Anthropology and psychoanalysis

What relevance does a psychodynamic understanding of culture have for anthropology? The central argument of *Anthropology and Psychoanalysis* is that, in order to explore the symbolic process and the nature of subjectivity, anthropology must transcend many of its traditional and self-imposed limitations and take on the lessons of psychoanalysis – in particular its explorations into the darker aspects of human experience.

In this collection of essays, an international group of anthropologists and psychoanalysts explore the interface between the two disciplines through the interpretation of culture. They reassess the project begun by Freud and point to new ways of seeing the relationship between the two disciplines and to new possibilities of collaboration. The first set of essays take their stand with George Devereux, who argued for 'complementarity' between the disciplines, regarding both as relevant to the task of ethnographic understanding but neither as being reducible to the other. It moves on to consider the Lacanian revolution and the implications for anthropology of this new synthesis between individual and society. A final group of essays explores the relevance of various types of psychoanalytic thinking for analysing ritual and symbolism.

The contributors' concern with issues central to modern anthropology – personhood, subjectivity, different modes of theorizing – makes *Anthropology and Psychoanalysis* essential reading for teachers and students of anthropology and a work of great interest to students of psychoanalysis.

Suzette Heald is Senior Lecturer in Anthropology at the University of Lancaster. **Ariane Deluz** is a Directeur de Recherche at the Laboratoire d'Anthropologie Sociale (CNRS), Paris.

Anthropology and psychoanalysis

An encounter through culture

Edited by Suzette Heald and
Ariane Deluz

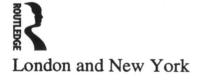

London and New York

First published 1994
by Routledge
2 Park Square, Milton Park, Abingdon, Oxon, OX14 4RN

Simultaneously published in the USA and Canada
by Routledge
270 Madison Ave, New York NY 10016

Transferred to Digital Printing 2009

Typeset in Times by LaserScript, Mitcham, Surrey

British Library Cataloguing in Publication Data
A catalogue record for this book is available from the British Library

Library of Congress Cataloging in Publication Data

Anthropology and psychoanalysis : an encounter through culture / [edited by]
Suzette Heald and Ariane Deluz.
   p. cm.
  Includes bibliographical references and index.
  ISBN 0–415–09742–8 ISBN 0–415–09743–6 (pbk)
1. Ethnopsychology–Congresses. 2. Social sciences and
psychoanalysis–Congresses. 3. Psychoanalysis–Congresses.
I. Heald, Suzette. II. Deluz, Ariane.
GN508.A65 1994
155.8—dc20
                                     93–44324
                                       CIP

Publisher's Note
The publisher has gone to great lengths to ensure the quality of this reprint
but points out that some imperfections in the original may be apparent.

Contents

Contributors

FLORENCE BEGOIN-GUIGNARD was born in Switzerland and studied psychology under Piaget in Geneva. She now practises as a psychoanalyst in Paris, has published extensively and is a member of the International Psychoanalytic Association.

ARIANE DELUZ was born in Lausanne and came to Paris to study anthropology under George Balandier and Claude Lévi-Strauss. She is directeur de recherche at the CNRS (Centre National de la Recherche Scientifique) and a member of the Laboratoire d'Anthropologie Sociale du Collège de France. She has done extensive fieldwork in both West Africa (particularly among the Guro and Youre of the Ivory Coast) and South America.

BERNARD DORAY is French and is a practising psychoanalyst as well as a technical consultant at the MIRE (Mission Interministérielle Recherche Expérimentation). He has also published (with M. Bertrand) *Psychanalyse et Sciences Sociales* (1988) .

IAIN EDGAR lectures at Northumbria University. He studied the use of myth, ritual and symbolism in a therapeutic community for his M.Phil. thesis in social anthropology and is currently completing his Ph.D. thesis on the cultural construction of dream interpretation in British dreamwork groups.

DINA GERTLER was born in Hungary. After the war she emigrated to Israel and later to France. There she trained as a psychoanalyst and wrote her doctoral dissertation under George Devereux. She now practises as a psychoanalyst in Paris and is a member of the International Psychoanalytic Association.

GILLIAN GILLISON was born in Canada and is Associate Professor of Anthropology at the University of Toronto. Since 1973 she has done field research among the Gimi-speaking peoples of the Eastern Highlands of Papua New Guinea. Her monograph on the Gimi *Between Culture and Fantasy* was published in 1993.

SUZETTE HEALD was born in Scotland and studied anthropology at University College, London. She has done extensive fieldwork in East Africa, most particularly among the Gisu of Uganda and the Kuria of Kenya. She is a senior lecturer at Lancaster University and published *Controlling Anger: The Sociology of Gisu Violence* in 1989.

L. R. HIATT is Australian and taught anthropology at the University of Sydney. He has done fieldwork among the Australian Aborigines and published *Kinship and Conflict* (1965), *Australian Aboriginal Mythology* (ed.) (1975), *Australian Aboriginal Concepts* (ed.) (1978) and *Aboriginal Land Owners* (ed.) (1984).

R. H. HOOK is Australian and graduated in medicine from the University of Sydney, later returning to read history and philosophy. He is in private psychoanalytic practice in Canberra, is a member of the International Psychoanalytic Association and edited *Fantasy and Symbol: Studies in Anthropological Interpretation* in 1979.

PIERRE-YVES JACOPIN was born in Switzerland and studied anthropology under Claude Lévi-Strauss in Paris and psychology under Piaget in Geneva. Later, he studied in Cambridge under Edmund Leach and did fieldwork among the Yukuna of Amazonian Colombia. He is now a fellow of the National Science Foundation of Switzerland.

HENRIETTA MOORE is British and studied anthropology at Cambridge. She is now a lecturer in anthropology at the London School of Economics and has done extensive fieldwork in Africa. She has published *Space, Text and Gender: An Anthropological Study of the Marakwet of Kenya* (1986) and *Feminism and Anthropology* (1988).

DAVID PARKIN is British and studied anthropology at the School of Oriental and African Studies where he is now Professor. He has done extensive fieldwork in East Africa, especially among the Luo and Giriama of Kenya. His books include *Palms, Wines and Witnesses* (1972), *The Cultural Definition of Political Response: Lineal Destiny among the Luo*

(1978), *Semantic Anthropology* (ed.) (1982), *Sacred Void, Spatial Images of Work and Ritual among the Giriama of Kenya* (1991).

CHARLES-HENRY PRADELLES DE LATOUR is French and studied anthropology in Strasbourg and in Paris. He has done extensive fieldwork in the Cameroons among the Bamileke and the Pere. He is directeur de recherche at the CNRS and a member of the Laboratoire d'Anthropologie Sociale. For the past 15 years he has also studied psychoanalysis at L'Ecole lacanienne de psychanalyse. He has recently published *Ethnopsychanalyse en pays bamiléké* (1991).

NIGEL RAPPORT was born in Cardiff and studied anthropology at Cambridge and Manchester. He now lectures at the University of St Andrews and has conducted anthropological research in England, Newfoundland and Israel. He has published *Talking Violence: An Anthropological Interpretation of Conversations in the City* (1987) and *The Prose and the Passion: Anthropology, Literature and the Writing of E.M. Forster* (1994).

GIULIA SISSA was born and educated in Italy and is now chargé de recherche at the CNRS and a member of the Laboratoire d'Anthropologie Sociale in Paris. As a classicist, her main interest is in the anthropological analysis of Ancient Greek culture and she has published (together with M. Detienne) *La Vie Cotienne des Dieux Grecs* (1989) and *Greek Virginity* (1990).

Preface

This book is based on a colloquium entitled, *Culture, Psychanalyse, Interprétation* held in Paris in July 1991 at the Collège de France. It was organised by Ariane Deluz and Suzette Heald and hosted by the Laboratoire d'Anthropologie Sociale. One of the inspirations for the colloquium was the cataloguing of the works and papers of George Devereux (1908–1985) at the Laboratoire by Ariane Deluz and Rupert Hasterok and it formed, as Deluz put it in her opening address, a 'reburial', a fitting celebration of his life and work and a laying to rest of his ghost. Our thanks go to Françoise Héritier-Augé for her hospitality at the Laboratoire and to the administrative staff, particularly Marcel Skrobek and Helene Monot, for their help.

We would also like to thank members of the colloquium whose contributions in the form of papers, comments and remarks during discussion are not fully represented in this volume: Patrice Bidou, Elizabeth Copet-Rougier, Vincent Crapanzano, Rupert Hasterok, Paul Jorion, Ben Kilborne, Adam Kuper, Mihaly Sarkany, Simone Valantin, Margarita Xanthakou and Andras Zempleni. Our most heartfelt thanks go to Pierre-Yves Jacopin for acting as scribe during the colloquium, for his summarising comments and for his important inputs into the discussions that went into the introduction.

The editors also acknowledge their gratitude to the following bodies for their financial assistance: Le Centre National de la Recherche Scientifique, la Mission Interministérielle Recherche Expérimentation, la Maison des Sciences de l'Homme, the Economic and Social Science Research Council and the Nuffield Foundation of Great Britain. In addition, we thank the following for giving their permission for us to reproduce copyright material: the Musée Barbier-Müller in Geneva for allowing us to make drawings of the statues nos 1007–1 and 1007–16 from their collection and to Doune Cesari-Tissot for making the drawings reproduced in Chapter 3; Oceania Publications for their permission to reproduce the quoted text in Chapter 11 and to Heinemann International for the text quoted in Chapter 12.

Translations from the French were done by Gordon Inkster, Monique Carruthers, Benedict Meynell, David Walker and the editors.

Special thanks go also to Therese Striggner-Scott for permission to use the figurines from Scott House, Accra in the cover design and to John Ziesmann for his photograph.

1 Introduction

Suzette Heald
with Ariane Deluz and Pierre-Yves Jacopin

This book brings anthropologists and psychoanalysts together in a common project, exploring the interface between the two disciplines through the interpretation of culture. It is based on papers presented at a colloquium, entitled *Culture, Psychanalyse, Interprétation*, held in Paris in July 1991 at the Collège de France, organised by Ariane Deluz and Suzette Heald. The colloquium took the form of anthropologists – French, British, Australian and North American – experimenting with psychoanalytic interpretations of their material. A group of psychoanalysts, also from international backgrounds, was then invited to comment on these interpretations. The book keeps the same structure in the hope of purveying some of the excitement of the colloquium and in order to point to new ways of conceiving the relationship between the disciplines and to new possibilities for collaboration.

The project begun by Freud on the psychoanalytic interpretation of culture has been largely ignored, when not explicitly rejected, by European anthropology, though even an unsympathetic commentator such as Edmund Leach (1958) could admit that the puzzle posed by a parallelism in interpretations has continued to fascinate. Today this fascination has new relevance as anthropologists have become interested in problems of subjectivity; in exploring the different conceptions of the self in a way which extends beyond the simple description of cultural difference to attempt to grasp something of the internal dynamic of a worldview. As the old reified view of society has been abandoned, anthropologists have shown a readiness to engage in a dialogue with a discipline which was at one time regarded as antithetical. At the same time psychoanalysis itself has moved on, with new interpretative methods which stress the importance of the interactive context and the temporal dimensions of symbolic formations. Symbolic complexes are no longer held to yield a determinate meaning, but rather seen as moving gestalts of signification. With both disciplines attempting to grapple with the radical indeterminacy of meaning, the time appears ripe for a *rapprochement*.

The analysts and the anthropologists came from a variety of traditions and nationalities but, above all, this was an Anglo-French dialogue, both the analysts and anthropologists working within their respective European traditions. In order to sketch out the lines along which such a *rapprochement* can take place, this introduction is divided into three sections. In the first, there is an attempt at a brief history of the relationship between European anthropology and psychoanalysis. The second considers the centrality of the fieldwork experience and leads to a comparison of the two situations of analyst and anthropologist in terms of the type of 'voyage' in which both are engaged. Exploring the nature of this 'voyage' and the epistemological issues it raises leads us to re-examine the contribution psychoanalysis can potentially offer for understanding the fieldwork situation as well as for the anthropological understanding of culture. Thirdly, we turn to the separate contributions to the book, and discuss the varied ways in which the sliding perspectives of psychoanalysis may support ethnographic interpretation and give insight into the lability of the symbolic process.

A HISTORY OF DIFFERENCE

Psychoanalysis has always been a literature of excess: it exceeded custom and reason, it overstepped acceptable scientific limits, it courageously explored beyond the prescribed authorities of modern thought. (Kohon, 1986: 75)

Perhaps the most notable feature of European anthropology and psychoanalysis over the last sixty years has been their estrangement. Initially, this was due as much to Freud's idea of anthropology as to the anthropologists' own concept of their discipline. Giving an ontological status to the phylogenetic evolution of humanity, in *Totem and Taboo*, Freud tried to apply the method he discovered for understanding the development of the individual psyche to society. But social history is not a simple reflex of the psyche and, since then, most anthropologists have remained rightly suspicious about psychoanalytic interpretations of anthropological data in terms predominantly of sexual symbolism. Despite this, the reception of psychoanalysis and its influence cannot be so summarily dismissed.

Indeed, somewhat paradoxically, anthropologists were among the first to apply and popularise Freudian ideas. Just as both Freud and Jung borrowed anthropological materials, in Britain, working still within the broadly conceived idea of the sciences of man developed in the mid-nineteenth century, Rivers, Seligman and, above all, Malinowksi had few hesitations in using psychoanalytic ideas to interpret their fieldwork. As

Fortes (1957) has remarked, Malinowksi welded psychoanalysis naturally into his functionalism, with his emphasis on the clash between culture and instinct and his penchant for a genetic interpretation of culture. The Trobrianders became the pointers to a new age of sexual permissiveness which Freudian doctrines were seen to promise. In America, the linkage of anthropology with psychoanalytic ideas was even stronger and Margaret Mead brought the convergence to an ever-wider audience. Yet the syntheses and applications that were here developed became increasingly marginalised on both sides of the Atlantic as anthropology came to define itself as a rationalistic and distinctive generalising science.

From then on the story has largely been one of divergence: anthropologists have seen themselves as dealing with cultural phenomena and analysts with the individual psyche, the one to be explored in collective settings, the other in the privacy of the clinical session. The relationship came to be seen in terms of a series of binary contrasts: collective/ individual, public/private, normal/abnormal. With each discipline sticking to its lasts, while there have been 'flirtations' and even maverick figures such as Roheim, Bateson and Devereux, there have been few systematic explorations of the interface between the two disciplines until recently, and, even here, very few and largely American.

Yet, despite the small numbers of practising psychoanalysts and the absence of psychoanalysis as a discipline from representation in universities, it has had a disproportionate effect on the very structures of our understanding of ourselves in the west. As Gellner writes, within a span of less than half a century, psychoanalysis has conquered the world, 'becoming the dominant idiom for the discussion of the human personality and of human relations' (1985: 5). Whether explicitly cited or not, it provides a perspective on the nature of the human condition which furnishes a set of background assumptions for all who have worked on the interpretation of culture. Whether 'for' or 'against', it is a perspective which has proved both durable and difficult to dismiss in its entirety. From lay psychologising to the critique of culture, the influence of Freud can be clearly discerned. As Ricoeur has argued, psychoanalysis provides a hermeneutics of culture which 'changes the world by interpreting it' (1979: 301). He cites Freud as one of the three twentieth-century 'masters of suspicion', who, together with Marx and Nietzsche, have questioned our illusions of consciousness and in so doing revolutionised our concepts of culture.

Yet, as has been pointed out, the different national traditions have interpreted the Freudian corpus in remarkably different ways, and this is reflected at least in part by its acceptance in the different anthropological approaches which have arisen in the United States, Great Britain and France. In order to understand the reception of psychoanalysis in these different traditions, we have also to comment on the different readings of the Freudian texts. To draw with a very broad brush, the Freudian tropos of ego, super-ego and id has been differently developed and elaborated, so that much American psychoanalysis has been seen to address itself to the nature and structure of the ego. In contrast, British psychoanalysis of the Kleinian persuasion has developed the deep moral implications involved in the creation of the super-ego, while the 'French Freud', as represented in the writings of Lacan, takes the unconscious as the true realm for psycho-analytic explorations.

America, somewhat to Freud's own surprise, from the very beginning proved extremely receptive to psychoanalytic ideas. As early as 1927, psychoanalysis was incorporated by the medical profession and its practice was (against the wishes of Freud himself) limited to qualified doctors. The American reading of Freud emphasises aspects of his work that have proved antithetical to some of the European traditions. Indeed, as Bettel-heim (1983) points out, the translation into English of the German, *das Ich*, *das über-ich* and *das es* into the cold technical jargon of ego, super-ego and id, had the effect of destroying their immediate personal connotations and converting them into a reified set of scientific concepts. Linked with its basis in the medical profession, this led to an over-emphasis on the mechanisation present in some aspects of Freud's thinking, just as it converted psychoanalysis to a utilitarian schema whose aim was 'cure'.

The individualist and hedonistic bent of Freudian theory in America has been seen as a clear ideological product of American capitalism (Craib, 1989). It ties in closely with the cultural values of American culture, with its essential optimism and the emphasis on personal freedom. The indi-vidual is seen as capable of affecting the course of his life, capable of changing him- or herself. This aspect has become more and more dominant in American psychoanalysis and its many offshoots as they have penetrated the general culture. The various theorists of what has been dubbed 'ego psychology', from Hartmann to Erikson, Fromm, Horney and Stack Sullivan, have been seen as developing an understanding of the conscious, self-directing aspects of the personality and its possibilities for 'adapta-tion'. In so doing, they underplayed the tragic aspects of the Freudian vision, associated with the forces of the id, of the unconscious and of the conflictual structures of the self.

If the optimistic strata in Freudian thinking came to dominate in America, as Hearnshaw (1964) has pointed out, a similarly purged and even more eclectic hybrid became conspicuous in the inter-war period in Britain. He comments that its compromises were perhaps typically British.[1] Yet, at the same time, a more pessimistic school of thought was developing in Britain through the work of Melanie Klein, and this has become increasingly influential in the post-war years, developed in various ways by Bion and Winnicott. In what is known as the 'British School' and as 'object-relations' theory, analyses have centred around the earliest infantile period, with the inevitable experience of conflict and the development of a moral sense arising in and through the social interaction of mother and child. Klein finds the genesis of moral consciousness in the 'depressive position', in the child's awareness of pain and suffering as an inevitable part of human relatedness. As the first stage of individuation, Rustin writes, 'the capacity for moral feeling is thus seen as a defining attribute of human beings' (1991: 20) and, unlike the super-ego of orthodox Freudian theory, not an external constraint, a source of guilt from which the individual may be liberated. Conflict is at the very heart of the theory, in the processes of splitting, of the projection and introjection of contradictory images and feelings which arise in interactional settings.

In France the neglect of Freud has been most noticeable, at the beginning reflecting the much more general neglect of Freud both by French intellectual culture and by the psychiatric establishment. The influence of psychoanalysis was subterranean, flourishing in the pre-war milieu of the café world of artists and intellectuals, particularly amongst the surrealists. A number of writers have commented on how the rationalistic basis of French thought, with its emphasis on human freedom, largely resisted psychoanalysis until it had produced Lacan, an 'indigenous heretic' whose structuralism and linguistic emphasis were resonant with the French Cartesian tradition (Hughes, 1966: 290; Turkle, 1978: 49). Even then, the influence was late, slowly developing in the 1950s and 1960s, leading to a positive explosion of interest in the 1970s which Turkle relates to the aftermath of May 1968. The interplay between the Marxists (especially Althusser) and Lacan was possibly decisive here, both because of the large part Lacanian analysts had played in the May movement and in the links that had developed between the left and Lacan. Deconstructionist, left- wing and unorthodox, psychoanalysis is not seen as the 'talking cure' but as a radical scientific discipline, a mode of research into the unconscious. Lacan's reading of Freud emphasises the first tropos of unconscious, preconscious and conscious, and the relations of meaning rather than those of mechanism. His most heated attacks have been on ego psychology: the ego is seen as the source of misapprehension, to be by-passed in the task of understanding the unconscious.

Just as the essential optimism of American culture led to an acceptance of a particular version of Freudianism and its popularisation, it likewise bred the same attitude in anthropology. Ruth Benedict's (1934) insistence on the malleability of culture and the plasticity of individuals is a good example here and, although she rigorously excluded psychoanalytic terms from her own interpretations, the idea of cultures being personalities writ large was there in the anthropology of the post-First World War period. Cultures were integrated like personalities – some more, some less. With the development of studies of national character and of culture and personality studies, closely associated with Ruth Benedict's colleague Margaret Mead, child-rearing practices became the key for many to understanding cultural values and patterns. Under the umbrella of cultural psychology a number of distinctive approaches arose, from the early configurationalism of Benedict, Sapir, Mead and Hallowell to studies of national character and modal personality associated with Kardiner, Kluckholm, Linton, DuBois, Gorer and Wallace among many others.[2] From the 1950s a more explicitly cross-cultural approach to the testing of Freudian-based hypotheses, as seen in the work of Whiting, Spiro, LeVine and Spindler, became more characteristic of American psychoanalytic anthropology, though increasingly marginalised in the context of American anthropology itself. Since the 1970s there has, however, been a strong resurgence in these approaches, uniting a fairly wide spectrum of opinion under the umbrella of cultural psychology.[3]

No such recognition has been accorded psychoanalysis in Britain despite the calls in the late 1970s that the time had come for a reassessment (Lewis, 1977; Hook, 1979). Hostility has remained the keynote in the relationship.[4] While this is not the place to review the 'phobic' relationship of British social anthropology to psychoanalysis extensively (see Lewis, 1977), some comment is due, for the antagonism to American cultural anthropology was equally marked. For the European traditions resting on Durkheim, the autonomy of the social and its irreducibility to the individual remained the basic tenet. With the growing distance between British and American anthropology, American cultural anthropology came to be seen as unrigorous and the development of culture and personality studies as reductionist and circular. Lewis is scathing in calling them the 'prostitution of anthropological ideas and material' (1977: 5). In this he was following a line of ridicule and calumny which had dominated debates in this field and which established hard lines between the social and the individual, the collective and the personal. The famous debate over Trobriand 'virgin' birth is an example here, and one cannot but have sympathy with Spiro who, in reviewing the literature on symbolic and structural anthropology in 1979, was moved to write:

> It used to be that one had to be a Freudian to believe that *nonsexual* themes in ritual and myth might possibly be viewed as disguised expressions of sexual concerns. It now appears that only a Freudian might believe that undisguised sexual themes might be expressions of sexual concerns. (Spiro, 1979: 6)

In France, the long separation between anthropology and psychoanalysis is perhaps more difficult to explain. For example, in the 1930s there began an important interchange between surrealism, psychoanalysis and anthropology. Parisian intellectual life brought together people like Betaille, Leiris, Lacan and Max Ernst. Later, during the war, Lévi-Strauss knew Breton and Ernst and their social circles overlapped in complex ways. The influence of surrealism, with its valuation of the unexpected mélange, the connection of otherwise disparate elements, can be traced in a certain poetic freedom which can also be discerned in the work of both Lévi-Strauss and Lacan, both revelling in the word-play and the pun. Yet, for neither is this mélange fortuitous: both drew for inspiration on structural linguistics and both put a model of language at the centre of their work. In each case the structure of the unconscious, whether in the individual or in cultural forms, is the structure of language. Despite these common and continuing intellectual roots, the written corpus demonstrates a history of largely independent development. Thus, while Lévi-Strauss claims Freud as a major intellectual influence, his theories of the human mind as the creator of culture have dealt with the psyche solely as an intellectual product, independent of psychoanalysis. For example, although his work on mythology may be said to cover the same terrain as psychoanalysis (as does his famous article on shamanistic cure, 1963a), it does so without engaging in debate or using psychoanalytic concepts. For Lévi-Strauss, it is logic not poetry which holds sway in ordering the unruly bric-à-brac of culture and its representations in mythology.

If this is true of Lévi-Strauss and his school, it is true more generally of French anthropology, despite its diversified, not to say schismatic, tradition. The organisation of the institutions for teaching and research and of the universities in Paris, together with the insistence on institutional and personal loyalties, divided anthropologists into mutually exclusive groupings. Each group has thus become associated with a different tradition. So, in the 1960s there were the followers of Griaule, pioneering the intensive study of cosmology through their long-term personal knowledge of their informants. Balandier's school put the accent on political dynamism, while the followers of Lévi-Strauss, like him, used structuralist perspectives to further the understanding of kinship and mythology. As in French village life, so perspicaciously observed by Wylie (1957), the French anthropologists make play with their differences and hostilities are open. By contrast, British social anthropology has seemed a more unified entity, tolerating a degree of non-conformity which, to follow the analogy, may well be seen in terms of English village life where attempts are made to avoid open conflict in the interests of an ideal of village identity.

The present engagement with psychoanalysis is then in no sense a simple one, since it involves dealing with different anthropologies as well as with radically opposed readings of the Freudian texts. The colloquium was notable for the presence of both Lacanians such as Pradelles de Latour and Bernard Doray and more orthodox psychoanalysts, affiliated to the International Psychoanalytic Society through their various national associations. Of these latter, both Florence Bégoin-Guignard and Dina Gertler practise in Paris, while R.H. Hook, who edited the 1979 collection of essays dedicated to George Devereux, joined us from Australia. All three are influenced by the work of Klein, Winnicott and Bion. The anthropologists also represented a variety of traditions. All the French anthropologists came from the Laboratoire d'Anthropologie Sociale established by Lévi-Strauss in Paris, while the English-speaking contingent was more diverse, drawn from various universities in Britain as well as Australia and Canada.

Nevertheless, as described above, all the anthropologists were working against a tradition in which psychoanalysis has been marginalised and in which the early anthropological engagement with psychoanalysis has survived in only tentative ways. Today, with the loss of old certainties and the basic questioning of the assumptions of the disciplines and their boundaries, the possibility of new modes of encounter is now open. So far this has led to relatively little serious intellectual engagement within Continental or British anthropology, in stark contrast to the position, say, in literary criticism or feminism. In the Anglo-French world it is still regarded as somewhat brave (not to say, foolhardy) for an anthropologist to stick so much as a hand up above the edge of this particular parapet. The postmodern experimentation with different perspectives and genres seems to stop short at this, and anthropologists are still likely to display an implacable hostility towards a tradition regarded as unscientific and reductionist.[5]

This is a pity for we no longer need to fight a rearguard action, detained by old battles. Psychoanalysis engages our attention for the sheer importance of the themes with which it deals – and its very intellectual disreputableness and power to shock. In showing each one of us in a light that we would rather not admit to, it is subversive to our commonsense view of things, dethroning our hope in the rule of reason and rationality. The unconscious is depicted as an arena constantly at war with conscious rationality, shattering our attempts to create plate-glass worlds for living. Even Gellner, never faltering in his belief in the triumph of reason, admits to the importance of its topics and reminds us that sexuality constitutes a problem for all societies: 'there is probably no aspect of life where the *pays réel* of the mind and the *pays legal* are so endemically at variance' (Gellner, 1985: 28). If, as anthropologists, we do not deal with this discontinuity we risk ignoring the darker side of human experience or, where not ignoring, anaesthetising it so that sexuality is transliterated into the rules and norms of kinship, violence into problems of law and war, dealt with on the political level alone. If we are to begin to grapple in a fuller and more rounded way with the existential problems of human life, then psycho-analysis with its intensive explorations into sexuality, fantasy and the inevitability of conflict, both intra-psychic and interpersonal, provides a crucially important perspective. Opening up issues which can hardly be approached in any other way, as Obeyesekere writes, 'psychoanalysis provides a much-needed corrective to a complacent worldview . . . by focussing on human suffering and pain and the roots of suffering in desire' (1990: 289).

Before further addressing the relevance of psychoanalysis for the inter-pretation of cultures, we turn to one other area where a psychoanalytic perspective is clearly relevant for anthropology: fieldwork.

VOYAGE

The very strength of anthropology – its experiential, reflective, and critical activity – has been eliminated as a valid area of enquiry by an attachment to a positivistic view of science. (Rabinow, 1977: 5)

The situation of the anthropologist in the field is fundamental to under-standing the nature of anthropological knowledge. Anthropology is voyage. It is not just a travelling in space from one destination to another, for the voyage also depends on the distance of the traveller. In his opening to *Tristes Tropiques*, Lévi-Strauss writes, 'I hate travelling and explorers' (1955: 1). This was a story of his field experience and the book is important not so much for its ethnographic detail as for the insight that we gain into his way of looking. The book introduces us to a philosophical journey. We understand the Indian in terms of his vision. Yet, as has been commented, this is a strangely impersonal book for an autobiographical account (Dumont, 1978). It is to this divorce of the personal and the professional, the fieldwork experience and the anthropological text that we now turn.

With Malinowski and Boas's invention of modern fieldwork, anthropology came to be based in and on practice. In becoming true travellers, anthro-pologists were plunged into the essential epistemological quandaries involved in the study of human behaviour. Initially, little of this was discernible in anthropological texts. The project of the Enlightenment, with its commitment to the canons of scientific rationality, still held and this led to the bifurcation of the ethnographic experience: one that could be told and the other that was consigned to silence. The public account took the form of the monograph, the detailed objectified account of the culture of a collectivity frozen in time and bereft of its author. The rest, the personal angst, if admitted at all, was committed to the private diary, rarely intended for an outside readership as was the case with Malinowski's *Diary* or, even more rarely, disguised in the fictionalised form of a novel, of which Laura Bohannan's *Return to Laughter* remains one of the most enlightening examples.

According to the canons of the discipline, fieldwork constituted an initiation, but it was one in which the idea of trauma was played down. Instead, it was conceived of as more like an initiation into a craft guild, where one learnt the craft through practical immersion and experience. Until the plethora of writing on reflexivity in the 1980s, there was virtually no commentary on how Malinowski's imponderabilia and confusions of everyday life were to be transliterated into the distanced style of academic discourse. The emphasis was on practical learning: through fieldwork the novice was to learn how an anthropological description was to be constructed; to learn what went into it and thus, by implication, how to interpret the monographs of other anthropologists. Through knowledge of one's own practice – the imperfect understandings, the ellipses, the difficulties of jumping from the specificity of individual happenings to the broad generalisation – the anthropologist learnt his craft, and hopefully improved upon it, part of the continuing and, as then conceived, cumulative tradition of anthropology.

This is not the place to comment further upon this process of rendering authoritative accounts (see Marcus and Fischer, 1986; Clifford and Marcus, 1986; Clifford, 1988). The aspect that concerns us here is their 'distance'. The accounts were de-emotionalised, presented as apart from the observer, who entered only as the independent witness, setting the scene and authenticating it. The I that was there was the eye of the camera. It was only this I which was relevant to the task of scholarship. With this we find the sharp delineation between the public presentation and the lived practice. And, in the same way, the anthropologist was expected to come back to join the community of scholars, now as an initiate, but bearing little trace of the experience in his or her own person. A parallel with Lewis Carroll's Alice suggests itself. Experiencing all the strangeness of the wonderland, Alice comes back essentially unchanged, the same rationalistic little girl we meet at the beginning of the story sitting on the grassy bank with her sister and with whom she awakes, back once more in her own world.

As long, therefore, as anthropology was seen as part of a scientific tradition, a methodology for gathering valid facts, the personal role of the anthropologist was effaced and psychoanalysis was inevitably marginalised. The task should not involve the self too deeply and the experiences of the anthropologist in the field were of no intrinsic interest. Returning from the field, many anthropologists of this generation found they had no one to talk to of their experiences; they were encouraged to forget, to regain the distance that had been 'compromised' in the field. Personal experiences were laid aside, to be anecdotally aired, maybe many years later, to amuse colleagues and students, part of the romantic lure of the discipline, of a story that could be confessed only in the pub, *after* the seminar.

Participant observation, then, with its polarisation of objective and subjective, left the anthropologist teetering unsteadily between the Scylla of pure objectivism and the Charybdis of 'going native'. It is true that some anthropologists of the mid-twentieth century, more involved with the epistemology of enquiry, had attempted to grapple with the imponderabilia of the anthropologist's subjective biases. Some, indeed, were intrigued by psychoanalysis, went to analysis themselves and, as Leach and Gluckman did, advised their students to do likewise before going into the field. Yet such advocacy stemmed from the perceived need to 'control' the erratic subjectivity of the anthropologist; self-knowledge was to facilitate a greater objectivity in the field, to turn the self into a more perfect observing instrument. In France also, many anthropologists went into analysis, both Freudian and Lacanian, from the 1950s onwards. We may suppose then that they were not ignorant of its message which destroys the illusion of any separation of the personal and professional. Yet, apart from a handful of famous texts (most notably, Leiris, 1946), this conjunction produced very little personal testimony.

It was for Devereux to explain the creative dynamics of the fieldwork encounter in its own right. In this, he was among the first to argue for the fundamental difference between the natural and the human sciences. Objectivity was not only a myth but a barrier towards a fuller understanding of the nature of the human person and society. Long before current concern with reflexivity and postmodern deconstruction, Devereux questioned anthropology's epistemology and sought to give 'involvement' a *positive* face. Though he remained resolutely realist in his approach, to this extent he prefigures much of what has been written in recent years.

Thus, it took Devereux, an 'outsider' and never completely integrated in the academic world, to formulate and elaborate the endless permutations of the anthropologist's situation. Born in 1908 from a German- and Magyarian-speaking Jewish family in what was initially Hungary but which became Rumania in 1919, he emigrated to France in 1926. From there, he left for the United States before the war and then returned to France in the early 1960s. Socially and politically displaced, it was among the Mohave while in his late twenties that he felt that he had discovered his real identity; an identity that was to remain throughout his life and which was given symbolic recognition in the dispersal of his ashes over Mohave land. It was their awareness of the unconscious factors in human life which made him conscious that they were 'psychoanalytically minded' and it was after this that he went into analysis himself. After the Second World War he worked as a psychoanalyst in Topeka in Kansas at the Menninger Clinic for war veterans, while continuing his work among the Mohave.

For Devereux, the two aspects of the anthropological dialogue, the aboveground and the underground, were always implicated in a dynamic tension where neither could be privileged. Like Alice, the anthropologist is in constant motion in a tunnel that links the conscious and unconscious and is the conduit from our world to theirs. This may also be said to be the means by which experience is transformed into knowledge, and 'Anxiety into Method'. This book, that Devereux worked on throughout the 1950s, was published in 1967 and contains in minute detail his reflections on transference and counter-transference, that is, the way the subjective projections of the anthropologist influence his understanding and the way, likewise, they interact with the unconscious projections of his informants. These reciprocities between the observer and the observed make the fieldwork situation fundamentally problematic, shot through with ambivalence, distortions, defence mechanisms and the trauma of the observer.

By this move, Devereux gave new importance to fieldwork as a method of social enquiry. Psychoanalysis taught him that anxiety was not something to be avoided but is the driving force which propels our intellectual questings. For the anthropologist, the necessity of complete involvement in fieldwork was the creative force in personal life and in the development of the discipline. By the same token, it meant constant vigilance for it involved the anthropologist working analytically with his or her involvement. In what amounts to a sophisticated modern reworking of the Devereux position, Obeyesekere (1990) distinguishes the three intersubjectivities 'at the crossroads where the cultural anthropologist must meet Freud if he is to undertake any kind of serious psychoethnography' (1990: xxi). These are, firstly, those of the cultural group studied, secondly, those involved in the anthropologist's relationship and reactions to that group and, lastly, his relationship with other audiences, most particularly his fellow anthropologists. In pursuing the second topography, Obeyesekere follows the same terrain as Devereux, though strangely without apparently noting this.

To bring interpretation to the centre of the anthropological endeavour is a way of acknowledging the subjective dimension of observation. The way forward is not to deny this problem, as the early fieldworkers did in their belief in the objectivity of facts, nor yet to go with postmodernist trends and deny any reality beyond the subject. The direction we would take is with Devereux, arguing that the anthropologist also conducts an experiment with him- or herself. The dialogue with the 'other' is both internal and external and has no natural conclusion. What is begun in the field remains for the anthropologist to work out in the rest of his or her life, both personal and professional. Kracke (1987) talks of the 'culture shock' often consequent on the return to one's 'own' culture which attests to the often radical dislocation in identity.

The voyage is a transformative event and its nature makes anthropology distinctive among the social and behavioural sciences. It also highlights certain similarities between the psychoanalyst's task and that of the anthropologist. Both forms of encounter involve the same kinds of questions in the relationship between analyst and analysed; both try to understand an other through interaction and dialogue. The multi-layed complexity of the analytic encounter and the sensitivity to context required comes out most forcefully in Hook (1979: Chapter 7). In acknowledging this, we do not want to underplay the important differences that exist in the nature of the relationship, in its perceived aim and in the theoretical apparatus used for interpretation. The anthropological encounter with the other is more varied, less 'controllable' in its nature and directed by different interpretative tasks.

A modern response to this epistemological dilemma has been to situate the anthropologist in the fieldwork experience and to write ethnography as a form of autobiography (for example, Rabinow, 1977; Dumont, 1978; Okely and Calloway, 1992) or as the kind of probing biography that Crapanzano demonstrates so well in *Tuhami* (1980). Yet, we would not argue that all psychoanalytically informed ethnography must take this path. Few anthropologists are trained to use their relationships and feelings as data in the psychoanalytic sense. The papers which follow illustrate a range of views, explicit and implicit on this topic. But most have taken the view that the anthropologists' prime concern is with cultural process and psychoanalysis offers an experimental perspective to engage with this material anew. For many, they are dealing with materials that they have worked on for many years, the papers revealing a long and often puzzling encounter with their subject.

THE PAPERS

Everyone has the responsibility of situating psychoanalysis in his vision of things. (Ricoeur, 1979: 323)

The anthropologists and psychoanalysts came from a variety of different persuasions and presented a number of different viewpoints. Nevertheless, one can distinguish three basic positions taken on the relevance and relationship of psychoanalysis to anthropology. The first is complementarist, seeing each discipline, after Devereux, as offering different kinds of insights into the phenomena under investigation. Anthropologists and psychoanalysts are here seen as working hand-in-hand, each elucidating cultural data from their own particular vantage points. The second position is informed by the Lacanian perspective which has resurrected the old Freudian project – though recast in radically different linguistic terms – in working towards a unified analysis of culture, a new synthesis of individual and society. The final set of papers also represent a more integrated endeavour. Relying in the main on more orthodox forms of psychoanalytic interpretation, the anthropologists here experiment with ethnopsychoanalytic interpretations of their data, transgressing the disciplinary divide.

The colloquium took the work of Devereux as one of its starting points and the first four papers are all exercises in the method of complementarity. Devereux is perhaps best known for his postulate as to the irreducibility of sociological and psychological explanations. Nevertheless, he held that they could both be applied to the same data and the interpretations that they offered would be mutually supportive. He illustrated this approach in his article on the notion of kinship (1978b) in which he took a case study from his psychiatric practice about a young man who found himself impotent with his fiancée who was also a cousin. This young man had previously seduced the sister of his best friend and his dreams revealed the necessity for the reciprocation of a woman. Devereux argues that this case reveals in a complementary way the necessity for exchange, paralleling Lévi-Strauss's (1949) sociological analysis. For both, the exchange of women between men privileges the relationship among men, revealing from Devereux's perspective a homoerotic element, while Lévi-Strauss is known for his dictum that men marry not so much to get a wife as to get a brother-in-law.

Each of these papers, like Devereux, uses a case study or text. Sissa takes the Oedipus myth while Deluz takes as her main text a song of the famous singer Bolia of the Ivory Coast which is based on a myth of origin of one of the Guro lineages and their failure to have a war fetish. Parkin examines the split between Islamic groups on the Kenyan Coast over the type of celebrations appropriate to celebrate the Prophet's birthday, while Rapport deals with the reaction of a group of Jewish friends in Newfoundland to a newspaper article which questions the reality of the Holocaust.

As a classical scholar and anthropologist, Giulia Sissa reviews a number of recent interpretations of the Oedipus myth. In so doing, she takes the classicists to task for their critique of the 'deep' interpretations of psychoanalysis. All interpretation implies going beyond the text and, in this respect, the Freudian hermeneutic is no different from those used by scholars of different persuasions. Coming to Devereux, she shows that he was always a man of many parts and gained a scholarly reputation not only in ethnography and psychoanalysis but also, in his final years, as a classicist. Somewhat ironically from the anthropological perspective, Sissa argues that in this particular case the 'ethnography' is misleading. Devereux argued that, in pursuing a psychoanalytic interpretation, the cultural ensemble could be used in the place of the free associations used in clinical work. However, in this case, the cultural evidence is too tendentious, based as much on the internecine disputes of classical scholars as on the supposed evidence. In arguing that Devereux was at his best when using his clinical perspective to articulate the symbolic associations raised by the actors in the Oedipus tragedy, Sissa's paper stands as a critique of classical scholarship rather than of Devereux's method as such.

Ariane Deluz takes up a classic psychoanalytic theme in dealing with the fantasised treatment of incest among the Guro. Starting with a myth, made famous in the oral tradition by a popular singer, the incest theme is found, though hidden, in the bisexual form of an incestuous father/ pangolin/father's sister. In interpreting these associations, the author turns to other myths and works of art. The theme of incest is shown to be evoked in many complex and subtle ways and these are, she shows, concordant with the system of kinship and marriage. Exchange is at the heart of the system, with men having to lose their sisters in order to gain wives. The complexity of the fantasies inspired by incest relates to the extreme ambivalence in intra-familial relationships which, in turn, relates to this system of marriage. Deluz's analysis is social, opening the way for, rather than offering, a 'complementary' account, and it is followed by a short postscript by Florence Bégoin-Guignard which indicates the lines along which a psychoanalytic account could be developed.

David Parkin admits to a greater agnosticism. Among the Islamic section of the coastal Swahili speakers of Kenya, there are different kinds of religious celebration. Some are seen as more 'Arabic' and restrained; othere are more 'Swahili' and allow for a greater freedom of expression. He notes that, among the latter, men dance in a way which is akin to women's dances of possession. This allows of a series of implicit oppositions between 'higher' and 'lower', Arab and Swahili, men and women. In this context, he follows the lead of Devereux to consider the role of the dance as expressing sexuality. Sceptical about explaining anything in terms of the symbolic association between dancing and the rhythmic movements of coitus, Parkin prefers a political interpretation based on a conflict between two Muslim groups. This is clearly a case where plausibility is given by the terms of a particular discourse – in Parkin's case, that of social anthropology – yet, as he maintains, no explanation is 'any other than speculative. Any human action can be attributed with an infinite number of meaningful associations', more or less compatible with each other.

If Parkin represents an agnostic position, Nigel Rapport argues the case for a linkage of perspectives. He deals with the possibility of a bridge between complementary perspectives in the form of a feedback mechanism, suggested by Devereux (1978a), in the idea of an ego-syntonic response. Here a single cultural event or movement operates to unite collectively a group of people, each drawn to it by a diverse set of individual motivations. In effect, such events 'harmonise' the collective and the individual. Rapport seeks to go beyond this vague hypothesis by demonstrating through a close analysis of the interactions of a set of Jewish friends how they negotiated their way to a collective response and forged a distinctive Jewish identity in a Newfoundland context. The importance of Rapport's argument lies in its identification of a particular type of rhetorical exchange – which he refers to as 'consiliar'- which allowed the individuals concerned to mobilise around a common collective trauma – the Holocaust – yet remain in other respects differentiated as individuals.

His analysis remains firmly social, but discussion of this paper raised the most divergences between the psychoanalysts and anthropologists, as is clear from the commentary by the psychoanalyst Dina Gertler and the subsequent reply by Rapport. Gertler gives far greater weight to the deep psychological effects of the Holocaust as a trauma which is transmitted from generation to generation. For her the micro-political dynamics are largely irrelevant and the group formation should be seen as a defence mechanism prompted by the newspaper attack, which not only awakens the unbearable knowledge of the Holocaust but does so in a way which constitutes a further denigration of the group members' ethnic identity. Gertler's own experience and the knowledge she has gained through her psychoanalytic practice leads her to the conclusion that the Holocaust is a non-assimilable event, an external persecution for the first generation and transmitted to the following generations as an internal structure in their psyche. The work of mourning is unending. She rejects the relevance of an ego-syntonic 'bridge'.

Rapport, in reply, takes up the important issue of the validity of different kinds of explanations of the 'same' event upon which Devereux's postulate of complementarity is based and further goes on to discuss the different conceptions of group and individual which inform his and Gertler's contributions. For Rapport the group does not unambiguously give an individual his identification – it rather provides an arena in which the individual may find or create an identity and this in a multiplicity of ways, of which the total merging of the individual in the group is one of the least likely. He is drawn to Devereux's idea that people are characters clothed by culture, but ultimately opposed to forms of psychoanalysis which appear to deny the validity of agents' accounts and conscious action.

The controversy aroused by this paper shows the legitimate divergences in perspective and reveals the degree to which each side may be 'shocked' by the other. The interest of the anthropologist in explaining current interactional events in terms of the present is here revealed in opposition to the analyst's reconstruction of them in terms of psycho-history, a return of the repressed. The idea of trauma, lying as it does at the heart of psycho-analysis, gave a certain emotive tone to these debates, striking as it did at the basis of the different methodologies of the disciplines.

This debate is carried on in somewhat different terms in the next section on the analysis of dreams, firstly by an anthropologist, Iain Edgar,[6] and then by the psychoanalyst R. H. Hook. Edgar is concerned with 'socially constructed meaning'. On the basis of his work with dreamwork groups, he looks at the metaphorical nature of dream imagery and its relationship with cultural metaphors. He is not concerned with the 'causes' of the dream but with the social meanings which participants are able to attach to them. His 'particular interest is in illustrating a process of transformation that is at the heart of dream interpretation and which sheds light upon the nature of our understanding of both self and world'. Thus, although these groups met in a semi-therapeutic setting, it is neither with therapy nor with the un-conscious that Edgar is concerned. Rather, his focus is on how meaning is achieved through dream imagery, a meaning which relates to current conscious daytime life. Psychoanalysis enters here not as a mode of analysis but as a cultural resource for the participants who readily picked up and interpreted dream imagery in sexual terms, a kind of 'dog Freudianism'. Perhaps this reveals most clearly Sperber's contention that 'exegesis is not an interpretation but rather an extension of the symbol and must itself be interpreted' (Sperber, 1975: 34).

This, though from a different perspective, might also be the position of Hook. However, Hook, as a psychoanalyst, by contrast sees the patient as using consciousness to gain access to the unconscious and for the purpose of thinking about it. Given the fracturing of psychoanalysis, he argues that 'the only way out of the present confusion of voices is to get back to [the] empirical base' of observations in the clinical setting. Hook takes the most significant develop-ment of Freud's thinking to be his introduction of primary and secondary process thinking and the role of phantasy.[7] While Hook argues that the opera-tions of mind can never absolutely be known, the transformation of an internal process through unconscious phantasy is knowable at least in part through dreams. As Freud demonstrated, dreams both conceal and reveal. What they reveal is not only content but the operation of the mind, communicating about, for Hook, its own 'defensive organisation'. But dreams do not only echo the structure of the mind, for they also use material from the external world and, in so doing, may either find reinforcement there in existing social institutions or create it to replicate themselves. He suggests that 'mythical and other ritual and belief systems and institutions may function in this way, facilitating shared identifications'.

What is essential to psychoanalysis, he argues, is the clinical setting between analyst and analysand and the processes of transference and the interpretation of transference. It is not the structure of explanation but the process by which it works that is the mark of analysis. Equally important, he argues, is the analyst's counter-transference – that is, what the analyst is able to perceive of the effects on him or her of the patient's transference. Thus, not only the patient's current life but the therapeutic relationship and setting itself form part of the context necessary to understand and interpret dream imagery.

As noted in the previous section, this sensitivity to context brings to light affinities between psychoanalytic and ethnographic methodology, even if the analyses ultimately point in different directions. For the psychoanalyst the awareness of the interactive setting is directed only partly towards the understanding of the current dynamics involved in the negotiation of identity and reality through social interaction. More important is the way transference gives notice of the significance of past emotive events informing the present interactions, which, by displacement on to the analyst and transfigured in fantasy, symbol and dream, are then opened up for renegotiation. For the anthropologist, with no similar narrative account to explain the origins of affect, the sensitivity to context is directed to the current diagnosis of a situation, to the on-going process of interaction and agents' conscious reflections on their situation, as is the case with both Rapport's and Edgar's accounts.

The third section of the book includes three papers which deal with the relevance of a Lacanian perspective for anthropology. Lacan, with a care for his reputation as an *enfant terrible*, might have been disappointed by the reception of his views at the colloquium. Three contributions set out the positive elements of a Lacanian view for anthropology and, while debated with some vigour, these expositions were met with curiosity and with appreciation of their authors for untangling the notoriously obscure prose of Lacan in order to provide an insight into how the theory might be adapted for ethnographic analysis. Yet, in so doing, in providing three readings of Lacan each systematising and developing an aspect of his writings, their projects may also be accused of being fundamentally un-Lacanian. As Vincent Crapanzano reminded the colloquium, the style is subversive because the message is; the play on words, the lacunae in the texts, the ellipsis and ridicule are part of the radical indeterminacy of meaning. Obscurity is part of the message; the writings follow the unconscious and resist lucid analysis.

Indeed, Lacan's reading of Freud highlights the radical split between conscious and unconscious, for the subject is taken to be incapable of knowing itself. The unconscious can never be known by conscious forms of reason. Psychoanalysis dethrones the Cartesian 'ego' in these terms and, for Lacan, the mistake of most other post- and neo-Freudian analyses is that they aim to reinstate the ego and the will as the master of the individual's destiny by giving it access to the language of the unconscious. For Lacan, this always remains opaque and the true object of psychoanalysis is not to provide a 'cure' but is 'an analysis of the unconscious which belies the subject's ego or consciousness' (Grosz, 1990: 27). Doray quotes Lacan in saying that the emergence of subjectivity cannot in Lacanian thought be reduced to 'a sociological poem of self-autonomy'.

Henrietta Moore's paper is programmatic in style and, taking off from the feminists' long encounter with Lacan, she, for the first time, tries to spell out what a Lacanian perspective, which drew together the anthropology of the self and the anthropology of gender, might imply for anthropology. She points firstly to the strange lacunae in the anthropological literature, whereby we have a burgeoning literature on the anthropology of the self, paralleled by that on gender, but these have largely remained as two independent literatures. Like other feminist writers, she finds the attraction of Lacan to lie in the *social nature of the theory*. Arguing, with Mitchell, that 'a person is formed through their sexuality' (1982: 2), she couples the idea that gender is central to the acquisition of personhood with Lacan's deconstructionist views as to the nature of gender itself. Throughout Lacan's work there is a questioning of any authority in the accepted notions of sexuality or psychic life: the biological essentialism found in Freud is disregarded in favour of a social and linguistic reading of the subject, a subject located thus in a particular historical situation.

Yet Moore, in reviewing the project, is led to agree with other feminist writers that the theory is still excessively phallocentric. As Bégoin-Guignard points out in her comments on the paper and on the Lacanian perspective, here again, the subject of psychoanalysis seems to remain that of 'a small Oedipal boy of 3 to 4 years old'. Why, Moore asks, should the 'phallus' always and everywhere be the key signifier of sexual difference? And why should we assume an inevitable binarism in the constitution of sexual difference? And why, given the ethnographic data, should we assume that the law of the father should be universal? In considering the positive aspects of Lacan's programme to be in its provision of a sociolinguistic theory of subjectivity, she again has strictures which relate to its excessive abstractness. We need, she argues, to move away from the structural level where language is seen merely as a system of signification, predicated on a system of differences, presences and absences, and move to the level of social discourse. It is at this level that the theory might speak to anthropology, taking into account the local views of the person and their cosmological and material situations. This is the direction in which modern feminist scholarship has moved. The cultural contingency of subjectivity, she suggests, will then be brought to the fore and this is the particular domain and expertise of anthropology.

Pradelles de Latour's paper is constructed along entirely separate lines in trying to give us an understanding of what a Lacanian analysis might look like when applied to ethnographic materials, in this case those of the Trobriands. The central concepts which he expounds are those of 'desire' and its relationship to the realisation of an innate 'lack', which the child experiences first in the 'mirror stage', which initiates the child into the dyadic structure of imaginary identifications and which 'lies at the base of the future reciprocity between the self and others'. Pradelles goes on to describe how the subject is established through the three Oedipal stages: in the original fusion of child with mother, in the mirror stage of mis-recognition of self in the imago and, lastly, in the Oedipal phase proper which serves to detach the child from its mother and the exclusivity of the dyadic tie to become a truly social being, focused on an object relating to the father. This is an act of both deprivation and displacement, initiating the child into the realm of the symbolic – of language and substitutions. Pradelles traces how these relationships may be seen to be constituted in Trobriand cultural forms. The identity with the mother is focused around her lineage and 'internal' ingestible nourishment while that with the father and his line represents the basis of separation and otherness. It is associated with articles of prestige wealth which favour seduction and sexual relationships.

Bernard Doray comes to the subject as a practising psychoanalyst sympathetic to Lacan and ethnographically informed. Developing from the contributions of both Moore and Pradelles, he takes on the task of explicating Lacanian concepts through ethnographic examples. Beginning with the mirror phase, he illustrates the processes of projective identification to underscore the Lacanian point about the impossibility of self-mastery. Human subjectivity resists the demands of conscious reason and the development of the subject is a continuous process of metamorphosis. Moving through the feminist critiques of Lacan's phallocentrism, he points to the complementarity of Lacan's vision with that of Lévi-Strauss (1963b) on social organisation. For both, dualism presupposes a necessity for a third term. The sexual, he argues, cannot be disinterred from the social.

The last three ethnographic papers in the volume, collected under the heading of 'working models', have a different focus. In these, three ethnographers adopt an explicit psychoanalytic frame to engage both with psychoanalytic theory and with ethnographic puzzles with which they have been involved over a considerable time. These papers perhaps fall more within the tradition of ethnopsychoanalysis, using the interpretative tools of psychoanalysis in an attempt to elucidate further data that they have analysed before. All these papers are concerned with ritual: Les Hiatt and Suzette Heald with male initiation rituals among the Australian Aboriginals and the Gisu of Uganda respectively, while Gillian Gillison uses her material on marriage ritual among the Gimi of New Guinea.

Hiatt's and Heald's papers in many ways form a complementary pair: both take a starting point in Freud's *Totem and Taboo* but they come to contrary conclusions about the role of initiation in resolving Oedipal tensions. The challenge taken up by the anthropologists here is the attempt to be specific about the particular conflicts figured in the ritual process. For Freud, the mother was the primary object of libidinal desire but the Oedipal complex was played out with respect to patriarchal forbidding. Indeed, Girard writes that 'the whole of psychoanalysis seems to have been summed up in the parricide-incest theme' (1977: 183). However, an important alternative model has also been developed in the anthropological literature which is more matricentred than patricentred. For example, Hiatt (1971, 1975) takes his clue from Roheim, especially Roheim (1945) in which he interpreted Australian myths and rituals as answering to separation anxiety and to providing compensation to the son for the loss of the mother. Similar themes have been elaborated in other recent work in New Guinea and Australia, where the extent of gender antagonism clearly raises the problem of the relationship between the sexes and the role of initiations in creating the cultural model of masculinity (e.g. Lidz and Lidz, 1977; Morton, 1990; Herdt, 1982). For some of these writers the issue, as with Bettelheim (1954), is that of female power and male envy. Unlike him, however, few have related this to the simple polarity of the sexes; most see it rather as induced by the strength of the mother and child bond in infancy and childhood. The making of men in such instances, it has then been argued, operates in terms of a dialectic whereby the boys are first feminised and then defeminised in order to be assimilated to male spheres of power. The rituals invite an interpretation as elaborate defence mechanisms whereby men both proclaim their superiority and arrogate to themselves the creative powers of women.

Hiatt now develops the lines of his earlier arguments through an examination of Stanner's material on Murinbata religion in order to consider more fully the relationship of fathers and sons. While questioning Freud's depiction of the 'primal sire', he nevertheless agrees that the initiation rites can be seen as strengthening the father and son bond, cathartically dissipating any Oedipal residues. The rites involve a decisive repudiation of mothers. A counter to this theme is found among the Gisu where Heald shows that mothers are centrally involved in their son's initiation and are presented in an entirely positive guise. Here, male circumcision does not appear to ameliorate tension in the father and son relationship but rather to intensify it.

With the classic lines of Freud's argument not 'working' in the Gisu context, a two-fold debate with Freudian theory ensues. Firstly, there is a problem about psychoanalytic interpretations in situations where the authority principle is weak in social life and there are no figures of unquestionable awe with whom to equate the Law. It is difficult to equate Gisu fathers with patriarchal forbidding. Nor is the alternative model developed for New Guinea and Australia immediately plausible, for the Gisu rite lacks strong patterns of sexual segregation, homoerotic rituals and fantasised images of female power. Indeed, the Gisu rites are notable for the way in which they create men, distinctively different from women, and, in so doing, valorise masculinity, but they do so in a way which draws the sexes together as much as setting them apart. Nevertheless, Heald argues that the stress on maternal symbiosis and the problems of individuation present an alternative mode of investigation. Drawing on the work of Klein and object-relations analysis, together with Lacan, Gisu circumcision here is regarded as an appropriate 'test' for the achievement of autonomy, marking, in the words of Wangusa, a Gisu writer, the 'journey we must all make'.

With Gillison's paper, the anthropological papers in the book come full circle. Returning initially to Devereux's suggestion that male homosexuality is an underlying basis for the development of marriage systems, she argues that he sold his theory short in considering it 'complementary' to a sociological one. On the contrary, she argues, this interpretation of marriage patterns, confirmed by her Gimi data, offers a radical critique of anthropology and one which can no longer be distanced by appeals to any 'superorganic' realm. She writes, 'If the human psyche includes an unconscious, and if the unconscious works in the way Freud described, then the findings of psychoanalysis bear upon every kind of activity.'

Arguing that an anthropologist should incorporate the insights of psychoanalysis by examining the unconscious dynamic in culture, Gillison examines the mythology and ritual surrounding the sacred flutes of the Gimi. The flutes which are used in male initiation ceremonies are normally forbidden to women. Yet, the same flutes are concealed among a bride's decorations as she goes to her marriage home. They are thus secret icons of the bride and indeed, from the male perspective, the flutes are constructed on a model of the female body and its sexuality. In women's myths, however, the flute – or its disguised equivalent – has a phallic significance and, in the marriage rite, refers specifically to the father's mythic penis. Thus, the marriage ritual takes on both incestuous and homosexual implications: the father, through making the flute for his daughter, not only recreates her in his image but also symbolically impregnates her. By taking the female perspective as well as the male's, the author gives a new insight into the workings of ritual secrecy and gender antagonism in this New Guinea context.

At this point it is necessary to comment further on the idea of complementarity. At one level, it seems an admirable doctrine, a licensed tolerance of other perspectives, allowing for a multiplicity of interpretative discourses. Each discipline is taken as having different vantage points, equally legitimate, each able to illuminate the matter under discussion in a mutually reinforcing, though non-reducible way. However, this maxim can be interpreted in different ways and it opened up a divide among the participants at the colloquium. For those – mainly the French – whose conception of the disciplines remains realist, the disciplines represent discrete strategic sites for analysis and the discourses can only run in parallel. The postulate of complementarity here provides a heuristic allowing for a dialogue but not for any questioning of the basic postulates on which the disciplines are based. For others – mainly the British – more influenced by the 'interpretative turn' in anthropology and psychoanalysis, the exercise provided an opportunity to reflect upon the claims made by the disciplines and their discussion therefore formed part of the current critical reflection on all modes of academic understanding. This allowed both for a more sceptical stance and for different ways of integrating the perspectives of the disciplines. Given the dilemma that results from the situation of both anthropology and psychoanalysis in a particular tradition of western scholarship, it is still possible to argue that anthropology's knowledge of other cultures and other constructions of the self gives access to data which can confront the universalistic claims of psychoanalysis. If this potential has been little exploited to date, it can point to a way of more fruitful co-operation, where the challenges are not to establish a complementary vision but to feed back creatively into both sets of disciplinary perspectives.

In his reflections on the issue of complementarity, we allow the psychoanalyst Hook to have the last word. In commenting upon the psychoanalytic themes in the last three papers and the relevance of the Oedipal dilemma, ambiguity and ambivalence, he now extends his earlier analysis of 'process' into the realm of 'content' in order to show how unconscious phantasy and culture reciprocally interact. Though disliking Devereux's term 'ethnopsychoanalysis' since it suggests the psychoanalysis of culture, he sees the future to lie in the development of an independent tradition, drawing on the findings of both psychoanalysis and anthropology.

NOTES

1   A similar spirit of British compromise can be seen in the division of the British Psycho-Analytic Society in 1946 into three groupings, the followers of Klein, the followers of Anna Freud and the Independent group which included Jones and Winnicott, drawing on the work of both Klein and Anna Freud (see Kohon, 1986).

2 See Bock (1980) for a useful summary of these approaches.
3 Much of this work is published in *Ethos* (the Journal for the Society of Psychological Anthropology) established in 1972. More recently, in the late 1980s, a new society for psychoanalytic anthropology was established under the rubric of the American Anthropological Association. It is also represented in a number of collections of essays (e.g., Shweder and LeVine, 1984; Stigler, Shweder and Herdt, 1990; Shwartz *et al.*, 1992) and in Spiro (1982, 1987), Obeyesekere (1981, 1990) and Herdt (1982), to mention only a few of the most notable recent works.
4 With the Malinowski/Jones debate over the interpretation of Trobriand family structure, Malinowski became radically hostile to psychoanalysis and this hostility was clearly felt in his seminars during the 1930s, as Fortes (1983) has recorded. It was not until the 1960s that Fortes and Turner were both able to brave, albeit *sotto voce*, the consensus and begin to explore psychological themes in their work.
5 A notable exception to this is Crapanzano, 1992.
6 Edgar's paper is the only paper in the collection which was not presented at the Paris colloquium.
7 We have followed the convention established in Hook (1979) in using the spelling 'phantasy' when the term is used by psychoanalysts and 'fantasy' when the concept is invoked by anthropologists (see also Hook, Chapter 7).

BIBLIOGRAPHY

Benedict, R. (1934) *Patterns of Culture*. New York: Houghton Mifflin.
Bettelheim, B. (1954) *Symbolic Wounds*. Glencoe, Ill.: The Free Press.
—— (1983) *Freud and Man's Soul*. London: Chatto & Windus.
Bock, P. K. (1980) *Continuities in Psychological Anthropology*. San Francisco: W.H. Freeman.
Bohannan, L. (1954) *Return to Laughter*. New York: Harper & Row.
Clifford, J. (1988) *The Predicament of Culture*. Cambridge, Mass., and London: Harvard University Press.
Clifford, J. and Marcus, G. (1986) *Writing Culture*. Berkeley and London: University of California Press.
Craib, I. (1989) *Psychoanalysis and Social Theory*. Hemel Hempstead: Harvester Wheatsheaf.
Crapanzano, V. (1980) *Tuhami, Portrait of a Moroccan*. Chicago: University of Chicago Press.
—— (1992) *Hermes' Dilemma and Hamlet's Delight: On the Epistemology of Interpretation*. Cambridge, Mass., and London: Harvard University Press.
Devereux, G. (1967) *From Anxiety to Method in the Behavioral Sciences*. The Hague: Mouton.
—— (1978a) 'Two types of model personality models' (1961);
—— (1978b) 'Ethnopsychoanalytic reflections on the notion of kinship' (1965), both in *Ethnopsychoanalysis: Psychoanalysis and Anthropology as Complementary Frames of Reference*. Berkeley and London: University of California Press.
Dumont, J.-P. (1978) *The Headman and I*. Austin, Texas: University of Texas Press.
Fortes, M. (1957) 'Malinowski and the study of kinship', in R. Firth (ed.) *Man and Culture: An Evaluation of the Work of Bronislav Malinowski*. London: Routledge & Kegan Paul.

—— (1983) 'An anthropologist's apprenticeship', *Cambridge Anthropology* 8: 14–51.
Freud, S. (1950 [1913]) *Totem and Taboo*. London: Routledge & Kegan Paul.
Gellner, E. (1985) *The Psychoanalytic Movement*. London: Paladin.
Girard, R. (1977) *Violence and the Sacred*. Baltimore, MD: Johns Hopkins University Press.
Grosz, E. (1990) *Jacques Lacan: A Feminist Introduction*. London: Routledge.
Hearnshaw, L. S. (1964) *A Short History of British Psychology, 1840–1940*. London: Methuen.
Herdt, G. (ed.) (1982) *Rituals of Manhood*. Berkeley: University of California Press.
Hiatt, L. R. (1971) 'Secret pseudo-procreative rites among the Australian Aborigines', in L. R. Hiatt and C. Jayawardena (eds) *Anthropology in Oceania*. San Francisco: Chandler.
—— (1975) Introduction to L. R. Hiatt (ed.) *Australian Aboriginal Mythology*. Canberra: Australian Institute for Aboriginal Studies.
Hook, R. H. (ed.) (1979) *Fantasy and Symbol: Studies in Anthropological Interpretation*. London and New York: Academic Press.
Hughes, H. S. (1966) *The Obstructed Path: French Social Thought in the Years of Desperation, 1930–1966*. New York: Harper & Row.
Kohon, G. (ed.) (1986) *The British School of Psychoanalysis: The Independent Tradition*. London: Free Association Books.
Kracke, W. (1987) 'Encounter with other cultures: psychological and epistemological aspects', *Ethos* 15: 58–81.
Leach, E. (1958) 'Magical hair', *Journal of the Royal Anthropological Institute* 88: 147–64.
Leiris, M. (1946) *L'Age d'homme*. Paris: Gallimard.
Lévi-Strauss, C. (1949) *Les Structures élémentaires de la parenté*. Paris: Presses universitaires de France. (English revised edition, 1969, Boston: Beacon Press.)
—— (1955) *Tristes Tropiques*. Paris: Pion.
—— (1963a) 'The effectiveness of symbols', in *Structural Anthropology*, Vol. 1. London: Allen Lane.
—— (1963b) 'Do dual organizations exist?', in *Structural Anthropology*, Vol. 1. London: Allen Lane.
Lewis, I. (ed.) (1977) 'Introduction' to *Symbols and Sentiments: Cross-Cultural Studies in Symbolism*. London and New York: Academic Press.
Lidz, R. W. and Lidz, T. (1977) 'Male menstruation: a ritual alternative to oedipal transition', *International Journal of Psycho-Analysis* 58: 17–31.
Malinowski, B. (1967) *A Diary in the Strict Sense of the Term*. New York: Harcourt, Brace & World.
Marcus, G. and Fischer, M. (eds) (1986) *Anthropology as Cultural Critique*. Chicago: University of Chicago Press.
Mitchell, J. (1982) *Psychoanalysis and Feminism*. Harmondsworth: Penguin.
Morton, J. (1990) Introduction to G. Roheim, *Children of the Desert II: Myths and Dreams of the Aborigines of Central Australia*, ed. J. Morton and W. Muensterberger. Sydney: Oceania Publications.
Obeyesekere, G. (1981) *Medusa's Hair*. Chicago: University of Chicago Press.
—— (1990) *The Work of Culture: Symbolic Transformation in Psychoanalysis and Anthropology*. Chicago and London: University of Chicago Press.
Okely, J. and Calloway, H. (eds) (1992) *Anthropology and Autobiography*. London: Routledge.

26   *Introduction*

Rabinow, P. (1977) *Reflections on Fieldwork in Morocco*. Berkeley: University of California Press.
Ricoeur, P. (1979) 'Psychoanalysis and the movement of contemporary culture', in P. Rabinow and W.M. Sullivan (eds) *Interpretive Social Science: A Reader*. Berkeley: University of California Press.
Roheim, G. (1945) *The Eternal Ones of the Dream: A Psychoanalytic Interpretation of Australian Myth and Ritual*. New York: International Universities Press.
Rustin, M. (1991) *The Good Society and the Inner World of Psychoanalysis, Politics and Culture*. London and New York: Verso.
Schwartz, T., White, G. M. and Lutz, C. (1992) *New Directions in Psychological Anthropology*. Cambridge: Cambridge University Press.
Shweder, R. A. and Levine, R. A. (eds) (1984) *Culture Theory: Essays on Mind, Self and Emotion*. Cambridge: Cambridge University Press.
Sperber, D. (1975) *Rethinking Symbolism*. Cambridge: Cambridge University Press.
Spiro, M. E. (1979) 'Whatever happened to the Id?', *American Anthropologist* 81: 5–15.
—— (1982) *Oedipus in the Trobriands*. London and Chicago: University of Chicago Press.
—— (1987) *Culture and Human Nature*. London and Chicago: University of Chicago Press.
Stigler, J. W., Shweder, R. A. and Herdt, G. (1990) *Cultural Psychology: Essays on Comparative Human Development*. Cambridge: Cambridge University Press.
Turkle, S. (1978) *Psychoanalytic Politics: Jacques Lacan and Freud's French Revolution*. New York: Basic Books.
Wylie, L. (1957) *Village in the Vaucluse*. Cambridge, Mass., and London: Harvard University Press.

Part I
Complementarity

2 Interpreting the implicit
George Devereux and the Greek myths

Giulia Sissa

However far back we go mythology has been interpreted. According to Plato in the *Phaedrus*, the Sophists created the philosophy of suspicion when they started to practise disbelief and to bring the narratives back down to earth. To say that Orythia was carried off by Boreas means simply that a woman died after being blown off a cliff by the north wind. What about centaurs, the Chimaera, the Gorgon, Pegasus and the other legendary monsters? Painstaking analysis could also 'set them straight'. The Stoics were subsequently to translate the whole of Greek polytheism into metaphysical terms relating to matter, form and natural phenomena. Plutarch, too, was to create a theory of symbolic overdetermination which Lévi-Strauss has praised, claiming that Plutarch understood the central principle of structuralism in recognising that a multiplicity of codes were interwoven in myth. Thus, early in the western tradition, myth became a narrative that could be understood only by going beyond its literal meaning. A refusal to take this step meant sticking to popular opinion, allowing oneself to be swayed by unquestioning beliefs.

The history of the treatment of myth in European philosophy and social science is a history of theories of interpretation, each positing a different yet coherent system of symbolic decoding: from Frazer to Ricoeur, from Max Müller to structuralism, and from the Cambridge historians of religion to René Girard. Here I am reiterating what everyone knows in order to establish from the outset the legitimacy of psychoanalytic interpretation as one going beyond the literal. When psychoanalysis turns towards mythology, using an interpretative technique that deciphers, decodes and reduces the phenomenon of narrative to a noumenon whose nature it claims to understand, no one should challenge the hermeneutic principle in the approach. It is surely the very opposite, not seeking to go beyond the living freshness of the story, that would be strange. A work that probably owes its success to such an unusual approach is Robert Calasso's *Marriage of*

Cadmus and Harmony, in which the author evocatively tells the story as a piece of unmediated mimesis.

An interpretative approach, sceptical about the actual words and syntax of the story, is thus certainly legitimate. However, it is another thing to ask whether it is also valid or, indeed, credible? We know how hard George Devereux had to fight in order to convince Hellenists of the scientific character of his exegesis. He wanted to lay the basis for a joint under-standing between philologists and psychoanalysts in order to give an entirely new and scientific understanding of Greece. I will try to show how his quest for truth gives value to his work and also the reasons why specialists in other areas have failed to understand it.

In order to identify the psychoanalytic approach, and more specifically that of Devereux, I will briefly compare the interpretations of the same story by different major commentators. We shall thereby see whether the psychoanalyst demonstrates the validity of his conclusions any better or any worse than other recognised interpreters. Of the narratives that have been subject to various readings, only one allows us to compare J. P. Vernant and Paul Ricoeur, Claude Lévi-Strauss and Jean Bollack, Marie Delcourt and George Devereux: the infinitely fascinating tragedy of Oedipus. The fact that these important commentators have all dealt with it is one thing; a more significant reason for studying it is that the non-psychoanalytic interpreters have expressly rejected Freud in a move to repossess the text distorted in *The Interpretation of Dreams*. An interest in Oedipus thus merges with a critique of Freudianism. There is also a third reason for turning to Oedipus: what is stated literally in it, and which Freud records as it stands, poses probably even more problems than that which can be found between the lines.

To recount the plot briefly. Laius and Jocasta, king and queen of Thebes, have a child whom they expose on Mount Cytheron, since the oracle predicted that if they had an heir he would kill Laius and sleep with Jocasta. The child survived. He was handed over to a shepherd by the ox-handler given the job of leaving him to die. The shepherd made a gift of him to his masters, Polybus and Merope, king and queen of Corinth. The child grew up believing himself to be the legitimate offspring of his adoptive parents. One day someone teased him by claiming that he was not really his parents' child. Upset by this he sought reassurance from his parents. They reinforced the lie by telling him he was indeed their son. In his anxiety he went off to Delphi to consult the oracle, and was told that he would kill his father and sleep with his mother. To escape this fate he resolved never to return to the parents he thought his own in Corinth.

Arriving at a crossroads he encountered a band of unknown men, who were in fact Laius and his retinue. After killing them in a quarrel over rights of way, he moved on to Thebes. This city was being terrorised by a monster asking the riddle 'which creature walks on two, three or four legs?' No one knew the answer until Oedipus solved it: man. By thus freeing the city, he was given the wonderful chance to rebuild his life: marrying Jocasta, ruling Thebes and having healthy children. Plague broke out. An oracle claimed that Laius' murderer was concealed in the city and must be driven away. Oedipus undertakes to discover the murderer and swears awful revenge. Sophocles' tragedy opens at this point when Oedipus commits himself in his ignorance. Soon after, a soothsayer hints to him that he is the murderer and that he is associating with people who are too closely related. Instead of immediately linking this to the Delphic oracle, Oedipus flies into a rage. So certain is he that his parents remain in Corinth that he begins to suspect his father-in-law and the soothsayer of a plot. He confides his suspicions to Jocasta. To reassure him, she proves how unreliable prophecies are by telling him that she was once told she would give birth to a son who would kill his father and sleep with her. To give the lie to this prophecy they had only to expose the son and, in any case, Laius had been killed at a crossroads by a brigand. Only now does Oedipus begin to waver. For the first time he wonders if there is a connection between the death of King Laius and the murder he committed at a crossroads near Delphi. He trembles at the thought of the curses he himself has laid upon the murderer. Yet he is still certain that his father is alive in Corinth. Only by bravely pursuing enquiries into the murder of Laius does he finally learn the truth. Jocasta hangs herself. He unhooks the corpse from the beam, rips off the clasp holding her garments and tears his eyes out.

It was precisely the direct and explicit nature of Sophocles' tragedy that struck Freud; nothing is repressed. He speaks of the:

> gripping power of *Oedipus Rex* . . . the Greek myth seizes on a com-pulsion which everyone recognises because he has felt traces of it in himself. Every member of the audience was once a budding Oedipus in phantasy, and this dream-fulfilment played out in reality causes every-one to recoil in horror. (Letter to Fliess, 15 October 1877, in Freud, 1954: 223–4)

The story as it stands transposes into reality a dream that is more or less repressed in the spectator. Later, in 1916, he was to ask: 'what help does analysis give towards a fuller knowledge of the Oedipus complex? That can be answered in a word. Analysis confirms all that the legend describes' (Freud, 1963 [1916]: 335). It is on these grounds, moreover, that Freud distinguishes Oedipus from Hamlet. In Shakespeare's play incestuous desire is shown opaquely.

But the changed treatment of the same material reveals the whole difference in the mental life of these two widely separated epochs of civilization; the secular advance of repression in the emotional life of mankind. In the *Oedipus* the child's wishful phantasy that underlies it is brought into the open and realized as it would be in a dream. In *Hamlet* it remains repressed; and – just as in the case of neurosis – we only learn of its existence from its inhibiting consequences. (Freud, 1976 [1900]: 366)

Thus where the spectator can readily recognise himself in Oedipus, unconsciously committing incest and parricide, it is left to the analyst to decode and interpret Hamlet's strange hesitation and hysterical symptoms.

Thus, in Oedipus, incest and parricide are narrated in all their unconscious fatality. Poetic language is no obstacle; on the contrary, it stages them and shows them being realised. This realisation or bringing to light, however, is compared by Freud to dream fulfilment. In their luminous transparency the narratives of antiquity allow a character to realise his desire and even the basic fantasy of the child. The narrative functions like any dream. What it unfolds is not merely a chain of discourse: it works out a symbolisation of desires, more or less deeply encoded. Thus the unconcealed presence in the narrative of the two troubling elements (killing one's father and marrying one's mother) is evidence for Freud of an act of symbolisation which refers to something beyond what is being presented. Behind the adventures of a character lies the unconscious desire of the child, of any child, of us all. This incestuous human desire is not in the text; it is in Freudian theory. The idea of the unconscious is not there either; it is hidden, encoded in the literary terms of blindness and destiny, and it too belongs to psychoanalysis.

Freud, then, draws our attention to what is perfectly obvious in the tragedy, but he does so in order to get sight of a phenomenon which, one way or another, needs to be understood, explained, explicated. Light is one way of representing (admittedly without repressing much but of representing none the less) something that the text ignores: the subject's desire. It is this reference to a desire that is unconscious – and therefore unspoken in every society – that embarrasses specialist interpreters. And from their standpoint they are probably right. The idea of unconscious desire belongs elsewhere. The question to ask, however, is the following: is a refusal to follow Freud into extra-textual analysis also a refusal to mistreat the literal sense of Sophocles' drama, or is it a rejection of psychoanalysis and its concepts? Listening to Hellenists makes one feel that they are concerned only with the respect due to the text or to the Greek reality (places where one finds no unconscious desire) and not with refuting psychoanalytic theory. They are challenging the application, the 'overlaying' of psychoanalysis, not psychoanalysis itself. But does not defending their own non-psychoanalytic approaches to literature and myth also involve applying to the surface of texts other interpretative methods that are, perhaps, no less damaging and abrasive? On closer inspection, the major commentators on Sophocles choose to go beyond what is said and treat the murder of the father and the marriage of the mother as signifying something else. It is only when faced with the thing that Freud naively took at its face value – the gripping drama of incest – that exegetists take their distance!

Delcourt (1944) devoted a fairly substantial study to Oedipus (*Oedipe ou la légende du conquérant*). As its title suggests, the author's intention was to see the hero's misadventures as centring around power and his relationship with his roots. Relying on a host of links between the earth and the mother's body, Delcourt argued that the real drama of Oedipus was tyranny. The same argument recurs in a much-read article by Vernant (1988) with the eye-catching title 'Oedipus without the complex'. Arguing from the symbolic links justified by the Greek ethnographic context, Vernant saw the drama as one about land and power.

Ricoeur devoted a chapter of his *Freud and Philosophy* to an exercise in dialectics based on the *Oedipus*. This demonstrated that the sceptical hermeneutic approach (interpreting as unmasking, reducing appearances to an underlying reality) must be accompanied by a further level of understanding as a way of recovering a meaning for oneself. He in fact claimed that Freud himself had set the same example. According to him, Freud began with a sceptical interpretation, decoding the tragedy by treating it as a sexual dream. In a second stage (a 'concerned' interpretation) Freud himself supposedly recognised that the tragedy was essentially a drama about knowledge:

> This interpretation no longer concerns the drama of incest and parricide, a drama that has already taken place when the tragedy begins, but rather the tragedy of truth. It appears that Sophocles' creation does not aim at reviving the Oedipus complex in the minds of the spectators; on the basis of a first drama, the drama of incest and parricide, Sophocles has created a second, the tragedy of self-consciousness, of self-recognition. (Ricoeur 1970 [1965]: 516)

Beyond the 'initial drama, which comes within the province of psychoanalysis', the philosopher finds 'the underlying link between the anger of Oedipus and the power of truth is . . . the core of the veritable tragedy. The core is not the problem of sex, but the problem of light' (Ricoeur, 1970 [1965]: 516–17).

Lévi-Strauss also chose the Oedipus myth for a sample structural analysis. The complexity of his approach warrants some discussion. In the first place, Lévi-Strauss considers the events occurring both before and after the story, from the ancestor Cadmus and the rape of his sister Europa by Zeus onwards. The fictional time-span of the narrative as it unfolds over several generations allows him to note the recurrence of related mythemes that can be grouped under four headings: the overrating of blood relations as evidenced in incest; the underrating of blood relations as evidenced in their murder; the murder of autochthonous monsters (and by implication the denial of human autochthony); the persistence of human autochthony. To reveal the relevant features of each group of related mythemes Lévi-Strauss brings in the ethnographic context (monsters = autochthonous individuals) and reaches the following conclusion:

> The myth has to do with the inability, for a culture which holds the belief that mankind is autochthonous, . . . to find a satisfactory transition between this theory and the knowledge that human beings are actually born from the union of man and woman. (Lévi-Strauss, 1963: 216)

There is no need to consider here the details of the 'American' interpretation. We need only note the distance between the mythical plot and the meaning revealed by analysis of the mythemes. Using the ethnographic context stressing autochthony (a theme that does not figure in the story) produces a markedly different result.

The last large-scale interpretation is that of Jean Bollack's (1977) four-volume commentary on *Oedipus Rex*. Bollack's starting point is the basic principle of hermeneutics as first expounded by Schleiermacher: understanding what an individual work means and grasping what the author intended to convey by use of signs, without falling back on any ethnographic context, or on any code or language whose impersonal and cultural connections could explain the symbolism found in the text. The common and generic language of the tribe in no way underwrites the meaning of the specific individual words used by the poet. The hermeneuticist must rise to the level of the poetic intention and grasp its uniqueness. Bollack actually treats the Oedipus story as a single entity (contained within a hermeneutic web) which reveals its full meaning by itself: Oedipus is born damned because his lineage has reached a kind of saturation point. 'Oedipus should not exist. Why? Because in Thebes, the home of plenitude and autonomy, any concentration of individual authority would endanger the world order. Oedipus is thus the instrument of Apollo's revenge' (Bollack, 1991: 21). Here too, however, we can measure the gap between what the story says (no mention of any particular vindictiveness on the part of the God of Delphi) and the meaning uncovered by the hermeneuticist. Bollack attributes to the Apollonian oracle a 'cosmological' purpose – re-establishing world order – that is nowhere explicit.

We can then sum up as follows: readers like Vernant and Delcourt find in the story a political meaning which makes the sexual element irrelevant. For them, incest means something other than sexual relations with one's mother, parricide means something other than the murder of one's father for a character who is the paradigm for it. Through a culturally contingent symbol (marriage with one's mother) a Greek poet sought to encode certain ideas about the relationship of the Greeks with the earth. He certainly did not intend addressing humanity in general, but only Greek spectators, for whom the connection between marrying one's mother and possessing one's native land would have seemed obvious, as the ethnographic context confirms. The correct interpretation is thus the one which respects what the text says in its own context and not in a void.

Ricoeur recognises the importance of incest only to show its insignificance compared to the 'real tragedy' whose nub is not sex but knowledge. Bollack emphasises instead the untimely birth of Oedipus; what follows is merely the sterilisation of his race. Lévi-Strauss does not decode incest and murder to reveal some other meaning, but the ethnographic context leads him to interpret the myth in terms of some insurmountable autochthony. We are thus drawn either towards an emphasis on the Greekness, or even the peculiarly Sophoclean nature of the plot (Delcourt, Vernant, Bollack), or towards its existential universality (Ricoeur). Lévi-Strauss combines both approaches by drawing on the Hellenist's erudition and the anthropologist's ability to compare.

I do not intend to pass judgement on the interpretations that I have outlined. I wish merely to show how non-psychoanalytic commentators face up to the question of validating their interpretations (by using the text, the ethnographic context and universal subjectivity) as a way of leading up to George Devereux. How will the psychoanalyst set about this same task? Freud read the text and sought to explain why, in itself, it had so striking an impact. He located any repression in the spectator and the latter's unease. Devereux, however, and this is why the comparison not only with Freud but with the others is relevant, found in it scope for his own style of interpretation. Indeed, he dealt with the Oedipus myth in the very lecture in which he laid down the rules of the method of complementarity as it applies to the Greeks.

His unpublished text is in two parts: the first is a plea to stick more closely to basic clinical principles when analysing cultural materials; the second shows that at a deep level self-blinding symbolically represents a castration, even though it may also refer to other kinds of blindness. The point that concerns us is the rigour of psychoanalytic interpretation and the relationship between what is said (blinding) and what is thereby symbolised (castration). Devereux begins by attacking those psychoanalysts who have gone in for a 'wild' analysis of literature or other cultural phenomena. In therapy, they would not (he claims) launch into interpretations involving deep symbolism without taking the patients' associations into account. Yet, when confronted by cultural productions, they allow themselves to draw directly upon a wealth of symbols allegedly codified once and for all. A direct reference to Jung makes the point of this polemic clear. It is precisely by reference to clinical procedures (and the requirement that the analyst should listen to his patient and follow up the individual symbolic connections in order to understand the particular shaping of symptoms and dreams), and therefore by reference to Freudian analysis, that Devereux urges the analyst to 'listen to' texts; to follow up the associations that culture and the ethnographic context build around every story and every myth. All of these relevant interpretations, all these bits of learned knowledge that one can gather together 'perform the part played by free associations when interpreting' (nd: 3). The analyst and the classicist therefore form the perfect team, the latter providing the knowledge to be analysed. With the Hellenist as the mouthpiece, Greece can unfold its symbolic and linguistic idiosyncrasies.

This opening proves the importance Devereux attaches to readings of the Oedipus myth and shows his wish to stress the logic of his approach. Devereux is extending to the study of a culture from antiquity (and for which only written information remains) the same interpretational method he advocates in his clinical treatments and in his ethnological investigations. If one compares the article on Oedipus with his article on 'Cultural factors in psychoanalytic therapy' (1980) one finds the general assumptions behind these multiple layers of shoring-up that, for Devereux, make up the human subject, including those whose existence is purely literary. His basic idea is that culture does not constrict or squash the individual, but rather that symbolic systems structure the subject and thus make him human. This structuring, moreover, does not amount to imposing uniformity or mimetic homogeneity; culture, on the contrary, offers individuals the means of differentiating and individualising themselves. 'In reality, culture expands the scope, range, variability, efficiency, and appropriateness of behaviour by substituting for massive and impulse-determined motility and affect-governed discharge a partial, specific, and narrowly goal-and-context-determined motility and affect discharge' (Devereux, 1980: 290). In other words, different cultures, with their varied types of encoding, support behaviour that is flexible and personal. By making sublimation possible they allow living desires to be expressed creatively, albeit in contingent and individual ways.

This rejection of subject/culture dualism, the idea that social rules and meanings shape and individualise people, provides an anthropological foundation for the complementary method. Just as the psychoanalyst is dealing with subjects who speak a particular language, belong to a certain kinship system, received such-and-such an education, all of which give form and content to their ways of being, so the reader-analyst finds texts that are already structured and stylised. And, just as the psychoanalyst must try to grasp the cultural and sociological codes of his patients – something which is all the more difficult when these codes are close to his own – so must he situate the fictitious characters who interest him within their own system of cultural references. He must turn himself into an ethnologist and a Hellenist, for as a clinician he is already concerned with culture, man being by his very nature a 'complementary' phenomenon, made up of universal drives and sublimated desires.

Even Oedipus, then, a figure whose archetypal character might seem to set him apart from cultural determinism, can be the subject of a complementarist analysis. The question that exercises Devereux initially falls within the realm of cultural encoding. Why did Oedipus poke out his eyes, why did he choose this particular means of castrating himself? Devereux's starting point is thus the symbolic equivalence between blinding and castration which he wishes to locate within a specifically Greek set of meanings. He wants to show that self-blinding is not an abstract disguise for self-castration, and thus why Oedipus' murderous hand strikes at his eyes and not at his incestuous genitals. The argument runs as follows:

1 By killing King Laius and marrying Queen Jocasta Oedipus committed an anachronistic deed: he behaved simply in the way anyone wishing to inherit power would have been required to act ritually in pre-Doric Greece, before the introduction of patrilineal transmission of sovereignty.
2 In making the king and queen also his parents the poet is representing the move from usurpation to inheritance.
3 Thus, in killing Laius, Oedipus is primarily killing a king and only incidentally his real progenitor. In any event, he is not killing his lawful or social father since Laius exposed him without going through the ceremony by which a man accepted his children.
4 Even if one retains the notion of parricide, it has been shown that Oedipus has already received the traditional punishment for parricides in the Mycenaean period – his ankles were pierced while he was still a child. Therefore
5 Oedipus has no need to punish himself for parricide and incest: firstly, because he was punished in advance, and, secondly, because the father he killed was first and foremost a king and from a social point of view (which is the main thing in paternity) he was not related to him.

Thus, Devereux argues, Oedipus was punishing himself for a different crime, and one for which his eyes are directly relevant, that of failing to recognise his parents. The young man who set out from Corinth knew that he was exposing himself to the fate depicted by the oracle; he should have avoided killing middle-aged men and marrying a widow older than himself. More than that, did he not possess a unique gift of clairvoyance that allowed him to tell people's identity by their age, as with the riddle of the Sphinx? Failure to recognise his biological parents was thus a false piece of non-recognition for Oedipus. Unconsciously he began to feel that he was the (real) son of Laius from the moment when he decided to avenge his death.

At this point in the argument Devereux feels the need to tone down the fact of non-paternity. One might well ask why, if cultural 'associations' lead one to deny any filial bonds, should falsely failing-to-recognise be, in the end, so serious that he should have to blind himself? If Oedipus' crime consists of a false failure to recognise his father and mother (with the complicity of unconscious desire) then his father must in some way be his father. Devereux then effectively modifies his first claim: the time when filiation required the ritual of *amphidronia* (accepting the child) was followed by a more patriarchal period when the bond of paternity was deemed to exist even without ritual and despite the exposure of the child. We find in the Oedipus myth a conflict between two cultural models. The greater part of the lecture thereafter expands upon the workings of the *acte manqué*, the way that from the outset everyone (Laius, Jocasta and Oedipus) acts to lock themselves into the fate laid down by the oracles. This, according to Pucci (1992), is in fact the most interesting and promising part.

One can now turn to the credibility of Devereux's interpretation. When it comes to validating and legitimating his approach, he is just as scrupulous as those other classicists who have dealt with the ethnographic context. But does that make him any more convincing? Unfortunately, his proof is weak precisely at the point where he relies on classical scholars. He overestimates their accuracy, their grasp of problems which are often dealt with only by conjecture or as part of polemical exchanges with colleagues. An individual's associations are likely to be more coherent than any historical reconstructions (especially for the pre-classical period). Thus, all the arguments about succession, filiation and the punishment for parricide must be treated with caution. On the other hand, Devereux is at his best when he analyses the unconscious intentions of the characters in the tragedy. He has most to say to us when he loses interest in the classicists' conjectures and allows himself to trace psychoanalytically the details of these figures from antiquity and the fascinating workings of their minds. The fragile status of complementary analysis in this case derives less from the use of psychoanalysis than from the hypothetical nature of the expert evidence.

BIBLIOGRAPHY

Bollack, J. (1977) *Replique de Jocaste*. Lille: Presses Universitaires de Lille.
—— (1991) Interview with R. Chartier and P. Lepape. *Le Monde* 28 June.
Calasso, R. (1993) *Marriage of Cadmus and Harmony*. London: Cape.
Delcourt, M (1944) *Oedipe ou la légende du conquérant*. Liège.
Devereux, G. (nd) 'A reappraisal of the self-blinding of Oedipus: an attempt at a rigorous application of clinical techniques to the psychoanalytical study of cultural materials', unpublished lecture given at Harvard University.
—— (1980) 'Cultural factors in psychoanalytic therapy', in *Basic Problems of Ethnopsychiatry*. Chicago: University of Chicago Press.
Freud, S. (1976 [1900]) *The Interpretation of Dreams* (S.E. 4–5). Harmondsworth: Penguin.
—— (1963 [1916]) *Introductory Lectures on Psycho-Analysis* (S.E. 16), trans. J. Strachey. London: Hogarth Press.
—— (1954) *The Origins of Psychoanalysis: Letters of Wihelm Fliess, Drafts and Notes 1987–1902*. London: Imago.
Lévi-Strauss, C. (1963) 'The structural study of myth', in *Structural Anthropology*, Vol. 1. Harmondsworth: Penguin.
Pucci, P. (1992) *The Construction of the Father*. Baltimore, MD: Johns Hopkins University Press.
Ricoeur, P. (1970 [1965]) *Freud and Philosophy*, trans. Dennis Savage. New Haven and London: Yale University Press.
Vernant, J.-P. (1988) 'Oedipus without the complex', in J.-P. Vernant and J. Vidal-Naquet, *Myth and Tragedy*. New York: Zone Books.

3 Incestuous fantasy and kinship among the Guro

Ariane Deluz

Among the Guro, the word for an incestuous person *trègyèzan*, 'killer of the earth' (i.e. of ancestors) is never uttered. Nor do we find any metaphoric usage; in my notes I have found only one metaphor relating to an incestuous person, which can be translated as 'the one who looks upon (the genitals of) a relative'. Thus, as in Sophocles, sight is endowed with power. Nor is incest ever referred to directly. In the discussions of marriages between those too closely related, they speak simply of 'miserliness'. Only the practicability of marriages is mentioned: 'so-and-so can marry that girl', 'he cannot marry this girl!' In this context, they describe genealogical connections which allow or forbid marriage between the two individuals, though, at the same time, no incest prohibitions may hold. The only absolute prohibitions are between primary relatives (father–daughter, mother–son, brother–sister) and even here, as has been mentioned, they are rarely referred to and, even when they are, only indirectly.

The official ideology of the Guro pronounces itself as favouring 'dispersed marriages': exogamy, exchange and generosity. But I am going to show that, on the contrary, there is a tendency towards endogamy, with its associated preoccupation with incest and incestuous longings – in other words, a complex of egoistic and repressed fantasies. This hidden aspect of Guro culture appears to be complementary to what is openly expressed and reveals itself through the seams of their social fabric, hinted at in their art and literature and in some forms of customary behaviour. In the following explication, a Guro song by the singer Bolia takes the central place, along the lines of the case study used by Devereux (1965) to outline his theory of complementarity and to show how a psychological account may be set against a sociological one.

THE GURO

The Guro form part of the South Mande linguistic group, as do the Dan, Tora, Mwan, Gagu, Youre/namane, Sokya, Gbeng and probably the Neyo in the Ivory Coast, and the Samo and other peoples in Burkina Faso, and yet other ethnic groupings in Guinea, Guinea Bissau, Sierra Leone and Liberia. Their home is spread over several administrative areas in the middle of the Ivory Coast. At the time of the French conquest (1905–12) the Guro were densely concentrated on the savannah and were more sparsely dispersed in the forested areas. They were primarily farmers, but also weavers, warriors and traders. In their habitat they took over from other people (who may be termed Proto-Mande) with whom they have partially fused and who are now encapsulated on their fringe: Youre, Wan, Mwan, Gagu and Sokya. Some Gagu, Youre/namane and Mwan lineages maintain that they previously formed part of a single people established on the savannah called Snanfla along the pre-colonial habitat of the Guo and Yaswa tribes; and archaeological remains such as stone sculptures representing the ancestor-earth to whom the Guro make sacrifice have been found there (Deluz, 1970).

Guro tradition has it that they came from the North with the Dan, from whom they became separated, although they still consider and treat each other as brothers. Their migrations may be summarised as follows. To the west, they have had a fairly long stay in the forest areas where some became permanently established (the regions of Daloa, Vavoua, Sinfra) and where they have frequently intermixed with the Bete; others moved off towards the savannah, some among them occupying part of what is now Baule country as far as Bouake; and they became concentrated in the Sub-Prefectures of Zuénoula, Gohitafla and Bouaflé. In the course of constant micro-migrations they slowly flowed back from Bouake and became infiltrated by the Baule with whom indeed they sometimes became assimilated. In short, many Guro were once Bete or Baule, just as many of these latter two are themselves of Guro stock. Today the Guro's neighbours are, to the west, the Bete, We or Gere; to the north, the Malinke; to the east, the Ayau and Baule; and to the south, the Baule and Gagu. The Guro and the small proto-Mande ethnic groups who preceded them thus stand at the epicentre of several ethnically, historically and culturally distinct peoples – the Mande/Malinke, the Kwa or Atlantic and the Akan.

Traditionally, Guro society was acephalous and the patrilineage was coextensive with a small village. These villages are grouped geographically to form 'tribes', in which some lineages play a preponderant role. Each of these tribes has a name and has certain economic, martial and also matrimonial functions, with marriage partners being sought among enemy lineages. Tribes are thus linked by complicated sets of friendly and hostile relationships, with a tribe which is a friend of your enemies not necessarily being your own enemy. This complex network also includes tribes of other ethnic groups such as Mwan or Monan, which are part of the system, having formerly been occupants of the northwestern part of the Guro habitat. What happened here, particularly in the northern part of Guro territory, was that, during the fierce resistance to the French invasion, many villages were burnt and their inhabitants were later regrouped. These new villages did not necessarily consist of a single lineage.

Guro descent is patrilineal. Assets and authority pass first from the elder to the younger brothers, and then to the eldest son of the eldest brother. This adelphic transmission has resulted in numerous splits and migrations. The system of kinship being of the Omaha type, the members of the mother's patrilineage (that is, the maternal uncles and also their sons and sons' sons) are all, for each generation, deemed to be your maternal uncles or fathers; and their sisters are considered as your mother. Descendants of your father's mother's brothers and of your mother's mother's brothers are treated as grandparents. And, symmetrically, the children of your father's sister (patrilateral cross-cousins) are your sons and daughters; and children of your grandfather's sister are your grandchildren (cf. Deluz, 1970 and 1993). A special word, *dini*, 'shell', designates the father's sister and by extension the father's mother's brother's son's daughter (FMBSD), the father's mother's sister's daughter (FMZD) and the father's father's sister's daughter (FFZD).

Residence is virilocal. For a woman, marriage is thus an exile, while, for a man, the presence in his lineage of wives from outside threatens to pollute the earth representing his ancestors. The marriage of a girl is sealed by bridewealth paid by the husband's family to her agnates, who then also use it for marriage. A wife may not be taken from a related lineage and bridewealth must circulate in the opposite direction to wives. This means that no woman may be given in marriage to someone of a lineage from which her lineage has already received bridewealth within a span of four generations. Marriages between affines may, in theory, occur only in two doubtful situations where the partners are on the edge of incestuous restrictions. First, a girl may be given in marriage to a patrilateral affine (e.g., her father's sister's husband) and second, a man may marry a matrilateral affine (e.g., a mother's brother's widow). The first is exemplary of a 'good alliance', but rarely occurs except to reclassify a 'bad alliance' undertaken with a person of inferior status, as will be seen later. However, a marriage with the widow of a maternal uncle is seen as a 'bad alliance' and very rarely occurs.[1]

THE SONG OF BOLIA

The above rather detailed presentation of Guro demography and kinship is necessary for an understanding of the sparse data on incest that can be found both directly and indirectly in oral literature and daily life. An examination of this in relationship to kinship norms, which it both expresses and contradicts, will demonstrate the kind of complementarity that is to be found among the Guro between the ethnographic phenomena and their fantasied ideological counterparts.

As I have shown elsewhere (Deluz, 1985), the ritual insults (*yunètan*) which are exchanged between the two tribal groupings Ma and Nya at the funerals of important men have, for the past fifteen years, moved beyond their esoteric origins and entered the public domain. This development has been furthered by a famous singer, called Bolia, who has refined some of these insults, and what they mean, in a poetic form. In his mouth these achieve an epic quality. In 1975/76 I recorded a song on which Bolia himself provides a commentary by way of *Sprachgesang*. My first recording of this text – the theme and Bolia's commentary are set out below – establishes this song as the founding charter for a clan. It evokes the well-worn theme of a primordial marriage between man and animal. Its relevance for the themes of this paper is in the multiple meanings of the word *zè* or *zèginè*, which the Guro use to designate the pangolin (*manis gigantea*).

The child of Na, the daughter of the Guo, named Yuro, has for father a pangolin.

If you go among a small group of the Guo tribe down there, you will find that the men react strongly if you speak of them as 'descendants of a pangolin'. Then, you should say that Bolia often speaks of it. Long years ago, when the earth was sweet [i.e., before the Europeans arrived] we black men fought only among ourselves. Yuro, a man of the Guo tribe, bewailed, as he lay prostrate before his dwelling. 'Everyone else has got a war fetish (*yu*) from its owner, but no-one has given one to me.' He thus laments and is the first to go to sleep, ordering his wives to feed the children. If war comes he will be killed [and there is thus no point in his eating]. When at midnight he rises to urinate, he sees in front of his house a metal chain hanging from the sky on which is fixed a *duan* [a word with the dual meaning of metal ring and watchman]. Yuro wishes to return into his house but the *duan* says to him: 'You complain endlessly that you have no war fetish, so let us go and make you one.' Yuro, the young Guo, thereupon climbs up the chain to the sky, and there his *yu* of the war is made and is put inside the belly of a male pangolin *zè*. Yuro, the Guo, then returns gently to earth down the metal chain. In a loud voice he there announces: 'I was lamenting that I had no master to give me a war fetish but now I have ascended to the sky to make one and this has been placed inside the pangolin.'

Now, one of Yuro's daughters was already grown and do you know where her father dug the pangolin's burrow? In the house where his daughters slept! And when he goes to his fields he leaves his daughter in the village so that she may watch over it. Everywhere, the story is told that a pangolin has its hole within that house. The men of Uebikohoufla come to see; the men of Byanwinefla come to wonder. All say. 'Is not this pangolin beautiful?' The men remain there and then, guess what, the daughter of Yuro is with child! When she is questioned, she replies: 'I sleep in the same house as my father's pangolin.' But, in truth, it is these men who came to see the pangolin who have got her with child.

On the day of the birth, Yuro's wife says to her husband: 'Leave. Your daughter is about to give birth and she has not spoken [i.e., stated the name of the father]. I am her mother and this birth we shall bear together.' Together, they bring into the world a single child, and when the father asks his daughter: 'Whose is he?' She replies, 'I know nothing; have I not told you that it is the pangolin's child?' The child is before them and Yuro declares: 'I placed my war fetish in the pangolin's belly. This pangolin whose pelt is a shell has put my daughter with child. Tomorrow I will kill it.' The pangolin hears him. That night he leaves his shell and climbs back to the sky whence it had come. Thereafter Yuro's war fetish is useless. The *yu* of the war is spoilt and woman is no longer kin to mankind.

The child grows. He stays with Yuro. When praising his name they call him 'descendant of the pangolin'. However, he was not born of the pangolin; he was conceived by man. Those who visit him, praise him as the 'child of the pangolin' but laugh quietly, saying with Bolia: 'This child was not conceived by a pangolin. It is the child of a man and the pangolin has been blamed for his birth.'

This insult deriving from the funeral rituals is far from clear. On the one hand, it is obvious to the Guro that the onlookers or admirers would take the opportunity to 'see' the daughter of the owner. Yet, this insult also recalls the promiscuity which is brought out in the psychoanalytic literature about incest where it is linked to deep loneliness. I think that the singer Bolia himself knows this. At this point in his poetic commentary, he introduces a paradox intended to mislead his listeners, but another explanation for the 'pangolin's child' is in fact contained in his text.

Bolia's secret truth is revealed in tribal art. Many years after having translated Bolia's song, I had the occasion to describe two fertility statues, one Mwan, the other Guro, in the Barbier-Muller collection: figures 1 and 2. Each of these shows, in its own style, a young pregnant woman: the aureoles of the breasts are enlarged, the belly protruberant, the upper part withdrawn, the buttocks in a characteristic posture. The girls look sad and

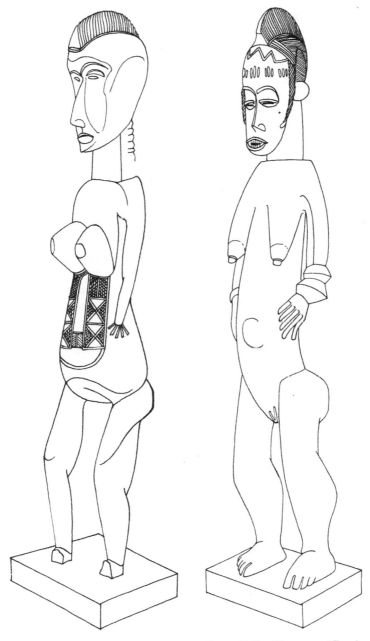

Figure 1 Fertility statue (Mwan)   *Figure 2* Fertility statue (Guro)
Source: Musée Barbier-Müller, Geneva catalogue number 1007–16

worried, not knowing what has happened to them. It was my assistant who drew my attention to their demeanour; he said to me that they attribute their pregnancy to the pangolin, as happens in Bolia's song. He expressed astonishment that I had not noticed that the word for pangolin, *zèginè*, can also be read as *zè* = 'that which is one's own', *gi* = 'within', *nè* = 'the child'; which signifies: 'he who puts a child within one who is his own' – in other words, 'the incestuous father'. It seems clear that these figures represent Yuro's daughter, whose child can now be seen as a consequence of her sexual relations with her father, for whom the pangolin stands as a metaphor. In the song, the daughter is thus, in coded form, speaking of incest.

Few of those who listen to Bolia's song today understand that the funeral insult aimed at the Guo (among whom are the families whose praise-name is 'pangolin') refers to the fact that their patrilineal clan was founded through an act of incest. What most believe is that the insult makes fun of them because the pangolin from whom they are descended is no help in war. The fact is, however, that the men of the Guo tribe are some of the best warriors among the Guro although they have no war fetish. The very name Yuro, *yu* = 'fetish', and *lo* = 'without', thus, 'lacking a fetish of war', recalls the story. Indeed, they are said to be so wicked and dangerous that, if they had a *yu*, they would be impossible.

Another explanation for their lacking a war fetish can be found in another of their myths of origin which I transcribed in 1958.

Banti is blind. His two sons are of different mothers. The elder, Bronon [eponymous with the Guro tribe called Bronon], is a farmer and he works for his father. The younger, Guo, is a hunter and regularly brings meat to his father. Banti promised his fetishes and wealth to Guo. When Guo is hunting, Bronon's mother brings Bronon disguised as Guo to Banti. Banti accordingly gives him his *yu* and when Guo returns, Banti can no longer keep his promise. Banti then says: 'My son Bronon and his children will be rich scoundrels, and thanks to their fetishes, they will have many children. My son Guo and his children will be few in number but they will be victors in all their wars.'

This story has an inverse symmetry to that in Genesis where Isaac by mistake gives Jacob, his younger son, the benediction he had promised to his elder son, the hunter Esau. This theme is not only found in the Bible but it is in the nature of a more general motif, a *Wandersagen*. In the story, the younger Guo hunter and warrior, whose name means 'jaw' (warrior), is here the opposite of the well-known African figure – the conquering foreign warrior who founds a kingdom. The father, Banti, is a figure who is recognised as at the origin of long migrations including that of some of the Bronon. Guo is probably the son of a younger and local wife. Perhaps this mythical fragment serves to justify the domination of younger brothers by their elders, emphasising the domination of the Mande Guro over the Proto-Mande Namane. In any case, the Guo have no need of magic to make war, since they are, eponymously, war itself.

History has indeed brought this fate to the Guo. The French considered them to be ferocious fighters against the conquest and, while some Guo lineages have spread into other tribes, very few Guo remain in their traditional habitat. In 1964, their seven former villages had been reduced to two lightly populated ones. In 1990, reassembled into a single village, they are poor and no longer possess their secret cults, which indeed they had to purchase. They are looked upon as the sorcerers and poisoners to whom strangers come for assistance. Meanwhile, the Bronon – descended from the other son of Banti – are both numerous and prosperous.

To return to Bolia, his pangolin story of incest occurs during that undefined period between the age of myth and the establishment of social rules. It is a time when sky and earth are linked by a copper chain. Later on, the break between earth and sky separates mankind from their distant and indifferent celestial God. Thereafter, men are linked to their ancestors whose village is below ground and stands in symmetrical opposition to the village of the living with which it communicates.

The term *duan* stands both for a ring sliding along a chain and for the watchman who takes Yuro to the sky. This word, however, appears in only one of the three versions of the story that I have collected. But *duan*, 'watchman' or 'spy', refers also to the *yuru* – 'sister's son', the intermediary between paternal and maternal lineages and thus of enemies in war and between death and life. From this arises the importance of the sister's son, who, as the indispensable go-between, digs his mother's brother's grave and makes sacrificial atonement to his mother's earth/ancestors if his mother's brother's wife commits adultery. Yet, he is a go-between whom each suspects of treachery and who is, more evocatively, deemed to be responsible for both order and disorder in the world.

In this context, we can see that the pangolin also plays an ambiguous role. It is a land animal which a man brings down from the sky and which he settles below the earth in the middle of his house. But the pangolin is also known for its feeding on underground termites' nests which are often called 'the clitorii of the earth'. In our tale, the pangolin enters as a pretext for the birth of a single human who will have few children. Yet, para-doxically, other Mwan and Guro women will come for their fertility rites to the women of this lineage. The pangolin sent away by the father, who is also his double and his human rival, leaves behind his shell and climbs back to the sky. The Guro never speak of its scales, but rather of its shell, *dini* – which is also the term for 'father's sister'.

Thus, in the first place, the pangolin recalls a kind of self-fecundation since it is usually talked about as a male animal known to adopt a passive defence against his enemies. In the story, it is itself made pregnant by a *yu* of war but it also makes the daughter pregnant, thus being in two ways 'he who puts a child within one who is his own'. At a mythical level, it provides a metaphor of undifferentiated sexuality and, at the pre-social level, it does the same for incest. After the birth of the child the pangolin abandons its shell on earth – could it be to protect its descendants? – and returns finally to the other world.

To go further, I now turn to one of the few known fragments of Guro origin myth, which explains their kinship terminology. As I have shown above, this terminology treats all members of the mother's patrilineage as fathers and mothers; and, conversely, the children of sisters as sons and daughters. The myth helps us to appreciate the many meanings of *dini* (shell and father's sister).

> At the beginning of the world, God brought to earth a pair of twins who married each other and produced a girl and a boy child, one after the other. These, in their turn, married each other and gave birth to two pairs of children who married both their fathers and mothers and also their brothers. Thereafter marriage between different generations was no longer repeated.

According to the elder who gave me this text, these marriages among different generations made it possible to diversify alliances and later, after several generations, to establish exogamous rules.

If we follow this myth, as depicted in Figure 3, a boy of the third generation could marry both his own sister and his mother who is also his father's sister. In the fourth generation, his children are divided into two groups: in one they are the children of both himself and his sister; in the other, they are the children of himself and his father's sister, who are simultaneously both his own children and his patrilateral cross-cousins. But these latter are also referred to as his sons and daughters. This is precisely the mark of Omaha kinship terminology. In turn, this Omaha tendency to telescope generations itself evokes the question of incest.

Although the myth tells us nothing about the transition to exogamy and thus of the necessity of the circulation of women, there is in Guro society a strong awareness of the exogamous break which affects all relations among women. Their simultaneous status as sister and wife is crucial. As a sister, a woman retains her ties with her own lineage; it is from this that she derives her fertility which is passed on by uterine descent. As a wife, she has duties toward her husband's lineage and gives birth to the children of his lineage but she is an outsider and suspect as the bearer of impurity.

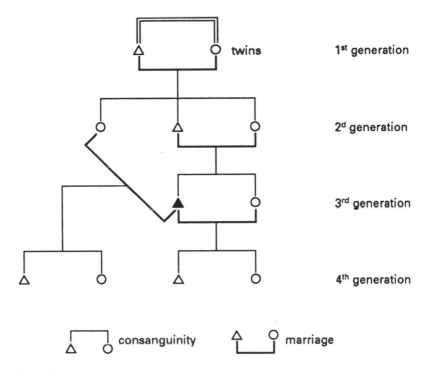

Figure 3

Socially, the mother and the father's sister (*dini*) are thus always in opposition. The *dini* embodies common lineage affiliation; she defends and protects her niece when the latter is subject to criticism in the family where she is married. The mother, on the other hand, calls attention to the perpetuity of an unnamed female line, which is a reality despite the fact that it is not socially recognised.

In Bolia's song, the *dini*/pangolin settles at the centre of the house and expels the father's wife who is mother and foreign to the patrilineage. However, she reassumes her place with her daughter in order to bring her to motherhood. This she does with her co-wives, thus delivering the child of the pangolin which represents both father and father's sister. Thus, to push this interpretation to its limits, in a paradoxical form, the outside mother becomes central to this endogamous complex of relationships.[2] Among the Guro, men are always excluded from the rites of birth which are the secret of women. Thus, Bolia can blame the women alone for this failure to kill the result of a known incest, a birth he finds so scandalous that it removes women from humanity.

Further, Bolia's tale draws a contrast between the relationship of the daughter with the father/pangolin/*dini*, which is one of fusion, and her relationship with the spouse/mother, which is articulate and uses words. In so doing, the mother restores communication and differentiation between father and daughter, by enabling the daughter to name, with a single word, both the genitor of her child and the act of incest. This episode fits with the practices of daily life where father and daughter do not speak to each other and where the mother/wife acts go-between.

When Guro men have been drinking, they often lament 'Ah, if only we could marry our sisters'. From this we can surmise that the kind of incest to which Bolia is referring relates to fantasies of incest between the father and his sister. This fantasised union results in *zèginè*/pangolin, a metaphor for *dini*, father's sister and shell, both sister and wife to her brother. As such she personifies in the myth the primordial marriages of brothers and sisters followed by a single cross-generational marriage, which thus establishes the kinship system.

The pangolin depicted as male also has bisexual attributes. He is a genitor pregnant with war, war which is synonymous with both exogamy and wealth. Yet, in effect, he aborts and leaves nothing on earth before making his escape to the sky. But the daughter, pregnant by this account by her father, by these means encapsulates all the strengths of the lineage, without the mediation of an outside spouse. The figurines previously described show that she is in a passive state. She has been impregnated by a bisexual being – at the same time, father/father's sister and a 'pregnant' male. Like a Russian doll, the figure is doubly pregnant, impregnated by a being itself pregnant.[3]

When the girl names the pangolin/*zèginè* as father of her child, she refers not just to a double but to a triple personality: a male vessel impregnated by war; an incestuous person who is her father; and the fantasised couple of her father and her protecting *dini*, the father's sister, protected by the shell of the pangolin. The pangolin is monoparous and likewise there is a single child born from the incest. This is the first-born child of a girl, who is, according to psychoanalytic literature, often fantasised by a girl as being her father's child, and is here dedicated to him. In this story, the child goes on to found a lineage. In fact, most Guro lineages are seen to originate from an act of transgression and, in this case, as has been noted, the child embodies all the strengths, masculine and feminine, of his lineage.

A study of the Mwan to whom the Guro are related confirms the attribution of bisexuality to the father's sister whom they themselves describe in a twofold manner: in the first place, the father's older sister, *zuru* in Mwan (a word which also means an antelope and is in turn a metaphor for leopard, both being animals of the Zamble cult); in the second place, the father's younger sister, *gwè* (a word which also means the royal doe, which is the metaphor for the Gu who is another personage of the Zamble cult). Among the Mwan, as later on among the Guro, the person of Zamble may be of either sex: when the mask representing the ancestor Zauli is present, Zamble is his wife and Gu is their daughter; when Zauli does not show himself, Zamble is the husband and Gu is his wife. The father's older sister may thus be 'wife' or 'father'; the father's younger sister either 'daughter' or 'wife'. The emphasis here is upon the bisexuality of Zamble and on the fertility represented by a red mark on the leopard skin upon the mask (Deluz, 1992).[4]

Again, another of Bolia's songs recalls a form of incest that is different from the one in the pangolin story. It concerns a wife who tries to persuade her husband not to use the bridewealth received for their daughter's marriage to marry a wife to their son. Instead she wants the husband to use the bridewealth for himself to marry a young girl who will become her junior co-wife. Such a wife is called 'daughter' in Guro terminology. In so doing, she will have direct power over a daughter in her household, and creates a semi-incestuous relationship between her husband and this 'daughter'.

As I have mentioned earlier, a young woman may be offered in marriage to the husband of her *dini*. Such a marriage is the closest not to fall under the incest prohibition. In fact it is rare and the Guro use it most commonly to secure marriages with or between their captives, who are referred to by kinship terms. At the sociological level, such a marriage of daughter with *dini*'s husband recalls marriage within the lineage and thus has similarity to incest. Incest creates a conjunction and short-circuits the kinship system.

All this, that is, the songs of Bolia together with the psychological inferences that we can make from the constellations of kinship among the cult personalities, constitutes a rich ensemble. Through it, it is possible to perceive incomplete projections, archaic fusions, partial objects, that is to say, an unconscious phantasmagoria. The way is now left open for the psychoanalytic account which follows.

PSYCHOANALYTIC POSTSCRIPT

Florence Bégoin-Guignard

The study above places us at the junction of two areas: the mind and society. Each has two sides. The mind separates and unites the latent and the manifest; society separates and unites the individual and the group.

In the first area Ariane Deluz reveals the prohibition on incest in Guro life as the re-emergence of the repressed. The breakthrough of the repressed is a mirror image of the primordial incest, the impossibility of returning to the maternal womb. It is buried in the forbidden word 'killer of the earth'. It is for this reason that the theoretically permitted marriage of a man with the widow of his mother's brother is considered bad; it represents the murder of the father. Conversely, other incestuous-like situations are openly institutionalised with minimal displacement and sublimation:

1 The marriage of a man with the daughter of his wife's brother allows him to accomplish easily a slightly displaced father–daughter incest.

2 The relationship of a man with his father's sister, *dini*, evokes a sublimated brother–sister incest.

3 The considerable authority of the *dini* over the household of her brother's son brings us back to mother–son incest.

In the second area, Guro society can be understood through Bion's (1961) work on 'group mentality', where the aim of communication is seen to be above all to maintain coherence in the group's life. As a member of this type of group, the individual will be allowed to express personal thoughts only in anonymous form and personal desires must be given up in favour of the group's coherence and homogeneity. 'The basic assumptions' that rule the group replace individual thinking ('minus K' in Bion's terminology) and they are an expression of the gregarious instinct. The language determined by the group's basic assumptions cannot be considered as primitive but as vulgar and 'trivialised' since it constitutes more a way of acting than a way of thinking. For instance, in the father-and-daughter relationship among the Guro, the language is always trivialised in this sense, except when the singer Bolia comes to the fore and dreams the 'myth of origin'.

NOTES

1 Without entering further on an analysis of marriage prohibitions, it is enough to say that the Guro system follows that discussed by Héritier (1981) as the 'cognatic sharing of prohibitions' (which for instance forbids marriage to a mother's sister's child, i.e., between matrilateral parallel cousins), in which she identifies the 'closest marriages' which still respect these prohibitions and the existence of strategies for bringing about a quasi-preferential exchange of wives between lines of descent (Héritier, 1981: 109–31).

2 The Guro do not venerate the pangolin as associated with their ancestors. Nor are the ancestors necessarily associated with fertility. Instead, their women seek help with their fertility from the old women of their grandmothers' lineages. The figurines are thus a metaphorical representation of the whole complex set of forces involved in fertility.

3 The girl's initiation rites also take up this theme of bisexuality (Deluz, 1987).

4 The changing relationships of kinship thus revealed and their links with emblematic animals such as the pangolin and leopard clearly recall the studies of

Douglas (1975) on the Lele and of de Heusch (1983) on the Lele and Hamba. In these Bantu societies, which are totally alien to the Mande group, can be found different combinations of the same cultural items to reveal different structural features.

BIBLIOGRAPHY

Bion, W. R. (1961) *Experiences in Groups*. London: Tavistock.

Deluz, A. (1970) *Organisation sociale et tradition orale, les Guro de Côte d'Ivoire*. Paris-La Haye: Mouton.

—— (1985) 'Histoire inattendue: insultes et récit épique', *Journal des Africanistes* 55: 187–202.

—— (1987) 'Social and symbolic value of feminine Knè initiation among the Guro of the Ivory Coast', in D. Parkin and D. Nyamwaya (eds) *Transformations of African Marriage*. Manchester: Manchester University Press for the International African Institute,

—— (1992) 'Le meurtre de la mère dans le culte du Zamblé, *Journal des Africanistes* 62,2: 183–91.

—— (1993) 'Affaires familiales et politiques', in F. Héritier-Augé and E. Copet-Rougier (eds) *Les complexités de l'alliance*, Vol. 3. *Économie, politique et fondements symboliques*. Paris: Archives contemporaines, pp. 139–64.

Devereux, G. (1965) 'Considerations ethnopsychanalytique sur la notion de parenté', *L'Homme* 5: 224–47.

Douglas, M. (1975) 'Animals in Lele religious symbolism', in *Implicit Meanings*. London: Routledge & Kegan Paul.

Héritier, F. (1981) *L'exercice de la parenté*. Paris: Hautes Etudes, Gallimard, Le Seuil.

Heusch, L. de (1983) 'La capture sacrificielle du pangolin', *Systèmes de pensée en Afrique Noire* 6: 131–50.

4 Islam, symbolic hegemony and the problem of bodily expression

David Parkin

The study of power relations is no longer primarily located in political anthropology, but extends significantly into the analysis of language use and psychoanalysis, as in the work of Derrida, Lacan and Kristeva. Attempts to link the conventionally political with the psychoanalytic have been few and mainly undertaken outside mainstream social anthropology (e.g., Legendre, 1976; Sagan, 1985). However, given the current view in anthropology of power as immanent in society and not the main or sole property of particular institutions, it is worth trying to relate apparently separate dimensions of the expression of power relations: put simply, do individual physical and sexual movements and gestures inform socio-political developments, or is the relationship the other way round, or is such a distinction ontologically false? I take a particular local-level case of Islam which I examine intensively in order to raise rather than answer this question.

While there is no single expression of Islam, there are certain general features which are commonly cited in the literature. A principal one is the prohibition on anthropomorphic and animal pictorial and sculptural imagery. Neither people nor animals, and only rarely plant life, may be represented. Instead, representations take the form of abstract designs in mosque architecture and of Arabic calligraphy. The prohibition may be assumed to stem from early Islamic attempts to suppress all previous forms of animistic worship (*shirk*) and of the deification of humans, as in the Christian view of Christ as consubstantially God.

There are many implications of this generally held prohibition in Islam at the local level. I will deal with only one here. This is that the ban on representing the human body pervades, I suggest, much Islamic thought on what is held to be appropriate religious and social behaviour and, moreover, results in hidden personal and interpersonal tensions which extend to conflicts of Koranic interpretation and, ultimately, to political contest.

I will take as my particular example the case of *maulidi* celebrations on behalf of the Prophet's birthday. As is well known, throughout the Islamic world there is a division between those who would wish to ban or restrict such celebrations and those who regard them as socially important and religiously acceptable. The argument for restriction or banning is that the Prophet himself condemned any public celebration of mortals, with only God deserving of such attention, and that many such *maulidi* include singing, the use of musical instruments, bodily swaying and movement and even dancing. The defenders of *maulidi* argue that, at the local level, such celebrations provide an important means of social and religious solidarity and, together with other so-called *bida* practices, give enjoyment and meaning to ordinary people's otherwise drab lives.

As Deluz points out (1979: 13), Devereux urged a kind of entry into the anxieties of the society under question through one's own anxiety as a fieldworker (1967). My own entry into the problem I address in this paper was not through anxiety but through a sense of frustration, bordering on occasional anger, at what, after many months in the field, became irksome restrictions placed on my own behaviour and constant admonitions to 'good' Islamic behaviour (including attending mosque for prayer and other occasions and speaking in a religiously appropriate 'arabised' form of Swahili). I was well aware that my being such an object of attention by senior Muslim clerics was a privilege, for it denoted my incorporation into and acceptance by the community of which I was a member and where I lived. But my recognition of my acceptance did not always lessen the frustrated sense of being constantly under surveillance.

It was through this experience that I think I understood the sentiment of many neighbouring non-Muslims (among whom I had worked on a previous occasion), who said that they could never enter Islam for fear of the restrictions to which they would become subject, including of their own frequent and prolonged dances which occur at funerals and other rites of passage, and at spirit possession seances, and their accompanying high consumption of palm wine and other liquor. For such people, this dancing and this drinking are essential pleasures which are interwoven with notions of amity, co-operative sharing, dispute management and political leadership and manipulation. As they themselves sometimes put it, there was here a conflict between Islamic rules or discipline (*masharti*) and the pleasures of a life free of such religion. Their own polytheistic religion, they said, created no such conflict.

It did indeed seem, when I looked back at my time among the non-Muslims, that I enjoyed there a degree of personal freedom that equalled and sometimes surpassed that of my own natal society, while later, among the Muslims, I alternated between marvelling at the camaraderie created through collective religious activities and railing inwardly at the religious discipline expected of us all. My own image of this latter ambivalence is of

Muslims desiring bodily freedom but subjecting themselves to collective religious constraint: they would argue about whether the body could or could not be used for rhythmic chanting and dance to the accompaniment of music.

I infer that the dispute among the Muslims themselves between those who oppose and those who defend the *maulidi* and other celebratory activities is, paradigmatically, of the same order as that between the non-Muslims and the Muslims as a whole. Thus, we can say that:

Non-Muslim 'bodily freedom': Muslim bodily constraint:: Muslim *maulidi* defenders: Muslim *maulidi* opponents (the 'purists, fundamentalists or reformists' as they are sometimes known).

Or phrased diagrammatically (based on Lévi-Strauss, 1979: 37):

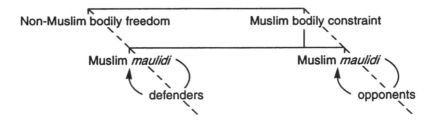

Under these conditions, there is a constant attempt by Muslim clerics to construct a scale of purity and holiness with regard to a whole range of behaviour. Yet, since purity is only ever a relational concept, there can never be a stage at which full purity has been attained. Hence, Muslim clerics are engaged in an endless pursuit in urging their congregation to acquire more parity through their behaviour. What may result, however, is the corollary: an endless attempt to restrict behaviour lest it be expressed in bodily symbolism. How successful is this attempt, and to what extent can we speak of bodily expression finding alternative personal and institutional venues outside religious activity?

In the area of the Kenya coast where I have worked, called Mtwapa, one significant consequence of the ceaseless attempt on the part of certain reformists to curb or alter the *maulidi* is to create a resistance among most local people, some of whom respond not by changing their heavily attended *maulidi* but by holding even more of them, often way beyond the month of the Prophet's birthday.

Can we, then, regard these proliferating *maulidi* as an expression of people's will to express their bodily freedom within Islam but out of the control of the more 'fundamentalist' of their clerics? In fact, it is not as simple as this, for, among the *maulidi* themselves, there is a distinction beween 'high' and 'low' forms.

The 'higher' *maulidi* are regarded as more 'Arabic' and the 'lower' more 'African' or 'Swahili'. Partly overlapping this distinction, though at times departing from it, is that between Wahabism and, for want of a better term, East African traditionalism. Wahabism takes the form of self-called Islamic fundamentalism originating in Saudi Arabia, that seeks to reinstate Islamic practice according to the Koran. The traditionalists are those East African coastal peoples who wish to continue with their customary practices, including the *maulidi* celebration of the Prophet's birthday, but whose practices are branded as *bida* (unacceptable innovations made since the Prophet's death) by the Wahabis.

The overlapping character of different *maulidi*, then, is juxtaposed to people's classification of them in oppositional terms. In other words, the flux and free exchange of characteristics is contrasted with their delimitation by fixed criteria. I argue that this is itself a way of opposing unrestricted and restricted uses of the human body in ritual, for, while so-called 'African' *maulidi* allow some bodily movement, 'Arabic' ones do not. I further argue that, while free bodily movement is associated with the non-Muslim origins of the Mtwapa people, constrained movement derives from Islamic teaching which forbids such an association. The proliferation and overlapping nature of *maulidi* threatens these neat distinctions and seems to be an indirect way in which people overcome dogmatic strictures and assert their own local and regional cultural distinctiveness. In doing so, however, they become part of a hierarchy of moral values which appear to inform their own judgements and personal views, indeed their social personalities. Are we entitled to suggest that the political and the 'ethnopsychoanalytical' are here linked and constitute common responses to the imposition of an ethos of purity? I hope to explore this question in this paper.

A BRIEF HISTORICAL CONTEXT OF THE *MAULIDI*

Let me begin with a few words on the recent history of the *maulidi* celebrations from the viewpoint of some key male elders on the island of Lamu, where the main Kenyan *maulidi* is held.

First, I give a brief account of the Lamu *maulidi* from a statement in the Lamu museum, probably formulated during the period before Kenya's independence in 1963, when the island was part of the British Protectorate, under the Sultan of Zanzibar. The current Lamu Museum education officer is the great-grandson of the founder of the present Lamu *maulidi*, and his views are in accordance with the Museum statement.

Maulidi is a eulogy on Mohamed's exemplary life. *Maulidi* is celebrated for several days during the sixth month after Ramadhan. The old version, called Barazanji Maulidi, was spoken in rhythmed prose, and it was read to a congregation. The new version, called Habshi Maulidi, is chanted, and the congregation respond in chant, swaying to the beat of rhythm instruments. These include tambourines, a small drum and occasionally a flute.

Habshi Maulidi was created by Habib Swaleh around 1900. He founded the Riyadha Mosque in Langoni, the southern section of Lamu Town. He was a likeable and sincere religious man and his form of worship became very popular with the people of the coast of East Africa.

As the Al-Habshi Maulidi grew in popularity, Habib Swaleh decided to have local dances performed to entertain the many guests. The first dance introduced was UTA, the coconut climber's dance, and it is still danced outside his house before Maulidi. UTA is also danced for weddings, circumcisions (as well as) *maulidi*. . . . Swahili weddings themselves are big social events . . . parties and processions take place for many days after the religious ceremonies.

A very full analysis of the Lamu *maulidi* is included in Moore (1977). As regards the above short text, I am not concerned with whether or not it is historically accurate, though broadly it probably is. Rather, I consider it as a statement which is regarded by local people as relevant to current issues. For some at least, it is a kind of charter. In it, and despite its innocuous style, we are introduced to some of the contentious issues that surround the *maulidi*. There is reference to chanting, swaying and the use of tambourines, in particular, and musical instruments generally. The event is referred to as a eulogy on the Prophet's life. Wahabi fundamentalists oppose such use of body and voice. They also argue that the Prophet himself abjured praising any man, including himself, for only God was to be praised. The founder of this new version of the Lamu *maulidi*, Habib Swaleh, is also reported as deliberately incorporating non-Islamic customary dances, one of which, that of the coconut climber, touches on what could easily be a sensitive area. Men climb trees either for coconuts or for palm sap. The production of coconuts, or the conversion of sap into vinegar, is perfectly acceptable to Islam. But the tapping of the sap as an alcoholic wine is strictly prohibited and is commonly attacked in *maulidi* sermons as a residual non-Islamic practice tantamount to a sin. Muslims are regularly castigated for allowing trees to be tapped for this purpose, even when the sale of the alcohol is to non-Muslims. In Moore's account, many other dances of non-Islamic origin are described, and, as in the above short account, there is the implicit view that, as regards dance, there is a similar festive element in both *maulidi* and weddings. One can well understand an

Islamic fundamentalist asking whether this means that the Prophet's birthday and an ordinary person's wedding are of equivalent standing. We see here the beginnings of the continuing and current conflict on the Kenyan coast between the Wahabi and traditionalists. Wahabism originates from Saudi Arabia and constitutes the teachings propagated by the supporters of Mohammed ibn 'abd al-Wahab of the early eighteenth century. Saudi Arabian oil money has in recent years enabled a small number of Kenyan Muslims to take up scholarships at colleges and universities in Saudi Arabia. They have sometimes returned with Wahabist proselytising orthodoxy based on close readings and interpretations of the Koran. By contrast, the traditionalists, or *bida* perpetrators from the Wahabi viewpoint, are traditionalist in the sense that they defend the practice of *maulidi* and other ceremonies as they have developed in the local East African Swahili context, with its undoubted incorporation of African Bantu elements. They do not claim that their *maulidi* practices are validated by the Koran, but consider that to celebrate the Prophet's birthday is a worthy religious act. They also say that it was through such joyous celebrations that Habib and his supporters could, at the begininng of the twentieth century, capture the interest of non-Muslim Africans living nearby, such as the Orma, who are now Muslim, and the Pokomo, a half of whom, living along the lower reaches of the Tana river, are nowadays Muslim, while the other half, living further away along the upper reaches of the river, incline to Christianity. (I shall describe later the other reaons which they give for continuing with the *maulidi* celebrations in their present form.)

Who, then, are the Wahabists and the traditionalists? In fact, there are very few self-professed Wahabists in Kenya. There are, however, a number of Muslims along the Kenya coast who have absorbed Wahabi views and who criticise the *maulidi* ceremonies and other kinds of so-called *bida*. These unacceptable practices include visiting and venerating the graves of religious leaders and other elders, holding extravagant funerals, supplicating and appeasing 'Koranic' and other spirits through shamans or direct possession, and showing respect for and kissing the hands of Sharifs, descendants of the Prophet.

The opponents of *bida* vary in the severity of their criticism. There are those few, especially recent returnees from Saudi Arabia, who wish to see the *maulidi* event as a whole completely eliminated. Others are less critical and wish only to reduce the ceremonial element, especially the chanting, singing and dancing. The latter are more numerous than the former, though still far fewer than the traditionalist majority who wish to preserve the *maulidi*'s present form.

Nor is the division between opponents and supporters of *maulidi* one that neatly coincides with ethnic differences. It is true that the Sharifs are drawn from peoples of Hadhrami descent. But not all Hadhrami support the *maulidi*. Hadhrami who have arrived in Kenya from the Hadhramaut in recent generations are the closest to being able to revive their links with and knowledge of Arabic, sometimes by working in Saudi Arabia. They may be decidedly lukewarm in their support. Peoples of Omani descent, on the other hand, generally do not accept the claims of the Hadhrami Sharifs to be descended from the Prophet and do not support the *maulidi* celebrations with which the Sharifs are associated. Finally, the Swahili themselves, particularly those who claim descent within what used to be called the Twelve Tribes, are generally in favour of the *maulidi* and other *bida*. Attaching themselves to these 'high-born' Swahili are the many other peoples who may variously call themselves Swahili by virtue of the fact that, as with the people of Mtwapa, this is now their first language. Such people, many of whom can trace some non-Muslim origins within their families, are also in favour of the *maulidi* and other *bida*. On the other hand, these latter are also prime among those who admire and aspire to the learning of Arabic, and so are open to external sources of persuasion.

The *maulidi* organisational picture is certainly complex. It is of Sharifs of alleged Hadhrami origin, though with roots in Kenya going back many generations, standing at the apex of a hierarchy of long-established Swahili families and of other Swahili, including some Muslims whose families have converted to the religion in recent times. This is a necessarily crude depiction, for even within a family its members may be split on the issue, but it is roughly correct.

For all the heated discussion that occurs, the current *maulidi* and *bida* practices are still very strong. Sheikh A. Badawy, the Lamu Museum education officer, and the great-grandson of the founder of the present Lamu *maulidi*, insists that, despite attempts by outsiders and those influenced by outsiders, there is no question of Wahabism or anything like it supplanting *maulidi*. During the turbulent period from 1977 to 1988, at least, he appeared to be correct.

We can illustrate the continuing strength of the traditional *maulidi* by comparing the influence on people of the two large mosques on Lamu Island. The old one was founded by Habib Swaleh in about 1889, a few years before he established the current version of the *maulidi*. It underwent renovation in the 1920s. Called the Riyadh College Mosque, it is 'owned' and administered by the Badawy family, of Hadhrami descent, and has been responsible for the religious education of a large number of maalims and imams throughout East Africa (see Lienhardt, 1959). It is a Sunni mosque teaching Sha'afite law, and the majority of East Africa's Muslims are of this persuasion.

In 1987 a large new mosque college was opened, called Swafaa, having been built through money donated by some Shi'ite businessmen from

Kuwait. The new college is actually administered by two men of the El Hussainy branch of the Badawy family, who 'own' and administer the older mosque. The two men split off from their 'brothers' to run the new mosque independently but in fact continue to observe the existing *maulidi* and other *bida* practices in much the same way as does the older mosque. Students attend both colleges from all over East Africa, with about seventy in each. The Shi'ite benefactors and at least some of the students at the new Swafaa college oppose *maulidi* and *bida*, as do the Wahabi. In addition, two reformist educational societies, namely the Ansaar Muslim Youth and the Muslim Welfare and Education Association, are reported to be opposed (although their main concern is in trying to integrate Islamic instruction with secular education). However, none of these sources of opposition has eliminated the basic form of the traditional practices, which, it is often pointed out, express the distinctive identity of Lamu and other indigenous East African peoples.

The defences made of the *maulidi* and other *bida* by senior traditionalists are often very powerful. For instance, Harith Swaleh, a prominent Islamic scholar of Lamu, spent fifteen years reading the works relating to Wahabism. He concluded that the doctrine went beyond a concern for stripping Islam of all innovations since the Prophet's death. For him, Wahabism is so opposed to all custom and therefore to a people's indigenous culture, that it leaves nothing in its place and ignores the community needs that are met through collective ceremony. He gives as examples, first, the Wahabi attempt to abolish the funeral ceremonial feast, or *hitima* as it is called. For a man to be able to share grief on such an occasion, as expressed in the phrase *mimi na huyu ni hitima moja* (we are of one funeral, i.e., we have seen this through to the end together), is both to assuage the pain and to express bonds of kinship or lasting amity. He gives as a second example the wish on the part of some Wahabi to ban the recitation by four elders of the four Fattiihya from the Koran on the occasion of a quarrel between two men in which one of them is injured. The Wahabi claim that the Prophet never in fact himself recited it and that it should not therefore be used in this sense. For Harith Swaleh, however, the abolition of this practice would remove an important means of reconciliation between enemies. By seeking to remove such customary practices, the Wahabi can, he said, 'become anything' for 'their philosophy is empty'. It takes away but does not reinstate anything of value.

On the whole the Wahabi public platform is limited, and the views of Wahabism occur more in texts, and in private conversation, than in open discussion. The essential aim is to 'purify' Islam of various trappings that the religion has accumulated since the Prophet's death. There is a special concern to eliminate lavish ritual focused on the Prophet, who is claimed to have denounced this himself, and on saints and the ordinary dead. In addition to Wahabi, there are some Omani who go so far as to claim that it is religiously forbidden (*haramu*) to celebrate the birth of anyone who has died. Wahabism also wishes to remove human intermediaries from people's direct worship of God. Man is joined to God by a direct line, and this should not be interfered with, which explains why the Wahabi contest Fattiihya recitations given by elders and the prominent role of maalims and imams at *maulidi* and other mosque events.

Inevitably, however, such moral absolutism becomes very difficult to define in practice. What is the line between the expression of modest respect for the Prophet and lavish adoration of him? Or that between merely remembering one's dearly departed and venerating the ancestors and saints? Even some critics of *maulidi* feel obliged to compromise. For instance, they may argue that it is improper to hold all ceremonies for the Prophet only on his birthday. They may urge instead that they be held at any time during the year, so reducing the intensity of focus on the Prophet and converting each *maulidi* celebration into one of thanking God for having sent him.

As we shall see, it is in fact the case that *maulidi* celebrations are held way beyond the month of the Prophet's birth, although they begin during that month. It is as if people accept the compromise entailed in staggering the ceremonies: they are for the Prophet but also for God. Whether or not such compromise, if it can be called such, really tempers Wahabi strictures is debatable. In the actual timing and conduct of the *maulidi*, however, it is clearly the case that there is a shading of one *maulidi* into another and an intermingling of different attributes.

Indeed, it is the participants and supporters of *maulidi* themselves who set up distinctions between them. They distinguish 'Arabic' from 'Swahili' *maulidi*, and collective from privately sponsored ones, as well as large from small. They also distinguish between *maulidi* verse which is long-standing, sometimes taken directly from the Koran, and that which is prepared shortly beforehand and even made up on the spot. Such criteria are often cross-cutting, so that a man or woman may be identified as the 'owner' of a *maulidi* which is not, however, privately sponsored by him or her but is long-established and paid for by the community of which he or she is the kinship senior or, in the case of a man, maalim. Here, it is the ordinary religious rank and file, more than the religious leaders of the *maulidi*, who make such internal distinctions. The maalims, imams, sharifs and sheikhs are much more likely to be concerned to defend and justify the *maulidi* institution as a whole in the face of Wahabi, Shi'ite and other opposition.

Thus, while religious leaders define *maulidi* for purposes of external representation, the ordinary people who attend them are more likely to see and evaluate the internal differences among them. The key distinction they make is that between 'Arabic' and 'Swahili' *maulidi*. The distinction lays the ground for a kind of contest to define who is a good Muslim. It may be remembered that at 'Arabic' *maulidi* participants tend to be constrained in their bodily movements and use of voice. In 'Swahili' ones there is less constraint. What, we may ask, is the significance of this contest?

Despite the inter-marriage and inter-union cohabitation that has occurred over the generations between Muslims of different ethnic groups, there is broad agreement as to who are 'Arabs', who 'Swahili' of the long-established families, and who Swahili-speaking Muslims and who non-Swahili-speaking Muslims of other kinds. Surnames are the most obvious set of delineators.

The reference to 'Arabic' *maulidi* tends to refer to one whose sponsor and/or main religious leader is a Sharif of Hadhrami descent bearing a name such as Al-Badawy, including El-Husainy, Al-Amudy, Al-Bory, Al-Mafarsy, Al-Khatib, Al-Ma'Awy, and so on, as distinct from people of Omani descent such as the El-Bakry, El-Busaidi and El-Mazrui. But the designation of a *maulidi* as 'Arabic' also refers to the likelihood that the ceremony will include recitations, verses and prayers taken from the Arabic rather than Swahili version of the Koran, and that the sermon may include summaries and refrains in Arabic as well as using a highly Arabised Swahili. To call it 'Arabic' may also, and perhaps most significantly, allude to the absence of tambourines and drums from the ceremony, and possibly of chanting and of the dances that sometimes occur after the formal conclusion of the mosque-based part of the event.

Those *maulidi* called 'Swahili' are thought of as reversing these characteristics: the main language is Swahili, Al-Farsy's Swahili translation of the Koran is used, the religious leader may bear a Swahili or Digo Muslim name, and the verses will be sung rather than recited to the music of tambourines, drums and flutes, and be composed for the occasion and perhaps elaborated there and then, with participants swaying, linking arms with each other and rhythmically bobbing up and down to the music, accompanied by various hand and finger gestures, which act as a prelude to dancing after the formal ceremony has been concluded. These are separate bundles of characteristics which are best seen as tendencies going in opposite directions.

Let me now describe some *maulidi* and show their distinctive and yet overlapping features, asking whether this overlap and its threat to neat classification account for tensions giving rise to moral pronouncements concerning 'correct' bodily usage. The following observations are taken from my field notes.

EXAMPLES OF *MAULIDI*

Mzee Athmani, the elder of the Mwando wa Panya Muslim community of fishermen in Mtwapa, observed that the Gunya, a Swahili group originating from Lamu, do attend the *maulidi* in the Mtwapa area but do not themselves hold any. They affiliate themselves to those held in their Lamu homeland. The elder described the *maulidi* in and around Mtwapa as mainly 'Digo' ones, each of which 'follows' a particular maalim of the area. For instance, Maalim Hassan, the maalim of my village and community, 'has his ancestors buried here, behind the mosque', and so he leads our Mwando wa Panya *maulidi.*

First, we shall attend a number of local *maulidi* held in Mtwapa catering for small groups of no more than a hundred people. They are usually called either 'Swahili' or 'Digo', the two terms used synonymously. Later we shall travel to Takaungu, Mambrui or Lamu for the large *maulidi* which are heavily attended by thousands of Muslims.

Just as most, though not all, local *maulidi* precede the major or national ones, so, among the local *maulidi*, there is also an order of precedence. In 1978, seven local, long-established *maulidi* were held, six of them on different dates between 9 and 19 February, and the seventh on 4 March, all during the month of the Prophet's birthday. The large, national *maulidi* of Takaungu was held on 22 February and those at Mambrui and Lamu were both held on 9 March. Others, in Mombasa, in Mtwapa and in rural areas of Digoland, followed these earlier ones, extending in a few cases well into the month of May. Thus, while there is an attempt to hold as many *maulidi* as possible within the month of the Prophet's birthday, there is also a tendency to go well beyond this month. This is partly explained by the alleged huge increase in *maulidi* and the emergence of new sponsors and new or refurbished mosques. But it is also explained by the wish on the part of sponsors and their communities to have a day which does not conflict with that of another *maulidi*. I do not know whether the fact that the major *maulidi* of Mambrui and Lamu took place on the same day reflected competition between these two old towns, or whether there were other reasons.

As one might expect, the local Mtwapa *maulidi* tend to be designated 'Swahili' and those of Mambrui, Takaungu and Lamu called 'Arabic', at least by the ordinary folk of Mtwapa. This is indeed a gross caricature, for, with every year that passes, local Mtwapa maalims try to up-grade the *maulidi* for which they are responsible. During the mid-1970s Middle Eastern money allowed for the building of new, and the refurbishment of old, mosques in Mtwapa. At *maulidi* held at two of these newly significant mosques in Mtwapa, major Muslim leaders, including some visiting from the Middle East, are invited to address the congregation. In this way, the two *maulidi* (at the Majengo and Shimo-la-Tewa mosques along the major road from Mombasa to Malindi) have indeed been up-graded, and are now spoken of as comprising a strong 'Arabic' element, for it is recognised that *maulidi* may combine this with 'Swahili' features. The effect has percolated down. For instance, a well-known Mombasa composer and singer of *maulidi* verse was invited to the 1977 *maulidi* carried out for my own small fishing community, shortly after he took as his second wife the daughter of our local maalim. He is of Hadhrami descent and referred to as 'Arab' by the local people. His presence and his marriage into the community were seen as a source of immense prestige.

This new development had the effect of introducing more formality into the *maulidi*, according to reports. Certainly, according to my own observations it contrasted strikingly with another local *maulidi*, which continued to be called 'Digo', i.e., an appellation that suggests even lower status than that of 'Swahili' in relation to 'Arabic'. The lower-order 'Digo' *maulidi* involved much chanting, singing and bodily movement to the music of tambourines, to such an extent that the men seemed to act as if possessed by divinity. By contrast, the newly up-graded *maulidi* was formally organised around the Hadhrami son-in-law, whose controlled and finely sung verse was the centre of attraction. It punctuated the mixture of Arabic and Swahili recitations and prayers in a precisely ordered manner, which had been rehearsed beforehand. At the same time it lacked the congregation of thousands, the microphones, loudspeakers, lights, large platforms and presence of numerous religious dignitaries of the more heavily 'Arabic' *maulidi* held eighteen days later at Lamu, which many of the Mtwapa people attended, despite having to travel a great distance.

There is thus a gradation of 'high' and 'low' forms making up the numerous *maulidi* which occur along the East African coast. They are described in terms of dichotomies, e.g., as being either 'Arabic' or 'Swahili', either private or collective, and so on. While the three major *maulidi*, and perhaps one or two in Mombasa also, remain supreme in relation to the myriad local ones, the statuses of these latter can alter.

A key feature of this distinction is the pattern of attendance. Broadly speaking, high-status Swahili and Arabs attend one or more of the few major *maulidi*. They only ever visit local ones if invited through a special connection, but this is uncommon. By contrast, low-status Swahili-speaking Muslims, including those often called 'Digo' or other Mijikenda Muslims, travel widely, both to the major *maulidi* and to local ones to whose sponsors they are connected through kinship and marriage. The people of my village in Mtwapa are an example. Together with other Mtwapa people, they hired coaches to Lamu and Takaungu for the *maulidi* there. They also, at different times, travelled in smaller kinship groups to other, more distant *maulidi* held by relatives. They look sideways, so to speak, among their own peers, as well as looking upwards to the higher echelons of Arab-Swahili society.

EXPLANATIONS

What, then, is the significance of the fact that 'Digo' and 'Swahili' *maulidi* involve chanting and bodily movement more than the 'Arabic' ones? I believe that there is an implicit connection between such vocal and bodily expression, on the one hand, and spirit possession dances and trance, allegedly of non-Muslim origin, on the other. From observation, again, the similarity struck me forcibly: the chanting, swaying, body movements and gestures by the men were highly reminiscent of those characterising women's spirit possession dances, except that in the latter there is spirit talk rather than chanting. In both cases, the impression given is of being possessed by 'spirit': that of God in the case of the *maulidi* and that of possessory 'demons' in the case of the cults.

The similarity between men's bodily movement in so-called 'Digo' *maulidi* and that of women's non-Muslim spirit dances is not that surprising, given the recency of conversion to Islam by the Digo people as a whole. They are thus close to their non-Muslim origins. It is true that, in this comparison, male and female roles have been reversed. But I see this as less significant than the continuity into Islam of the idea of human bodily possession by an extra-human spiritual force, with the result that the idiom of bodily expression is preserved. But it is not only these recently converted Digo who can be said to be closely connected to these bodily reminiscences of polytheism (*ushirikina* or *shirk*). It is a perennial theme of many *maulidi* sermons of whatever level: the congregation is urged by the preacher not to depart from the ways of Islam. They must not drink alcohol, consult shamans and their spirits, seek the help of nature spirits, venerate ancestors nor spend time and money on funerals, as is the custom among the non-Muslim Mijikenda.

I suggest, therefore, that, in arguing against such non-Muslim 'impurities', including women's spirit possession dances, the *maulidi* religious leaders are in effect voicing the same underlying objections as the Wahabi who oppose *maulidi* as a whole. The Wahabi, after all, also focus on the use of musical instruments, singing and dancing as being unacceptable to their version of Islam. In other words, both those maalims who defend *maulidi* and those Wahabi and others who oppose them hover around an objection to the use of individual bodies and voices: maalims oppose spirit dances among women; and Wahabi criticise men's *maulidi* music, song and dance.

But what is it that the religious leaders object to when they try to dissuade members of a Muslim congregation from expressing themselves individually through body and voice? Here we encounter the crux of analysis. For there are a number of interpretations that may be attempted. First, there is what I will call the political explanation. This is that the use of body and voice expresses an individuality which the religious leaders oppose on account of its threat to their own authority. By this argument, the lower-status Muslims, being the most vociferous and bodily active at their *maulidi*, are also the most individualistic and so the most potentially challenging to religious authority which seeks to control individualism before the absolute authority of God. To this extent, such people seem to be religious rebels asserting their own pre-Islamic customary selfhood and identity. Yet, they do not appear to see things this way. They do, after all, seek to raise their status closer to that of higher-order Muslims who see themselves as distant from any non-Muslim origins and who comply with religious authority and subordinate their individuality to it. Is this a curious case of false consciousness on the part of an under-class? Or is it more simply a case of people who, given the chance, will anywhere wish to express religious enthusiasm through dance and song rather than bodily constraint and text?

This latter suggestion takes us away from political explanation to one based on a notion of human 'need', namely that religious expression will tend to take exuberant bodily forms. In fact, there are too many obverse cases without human bodily movement elsewhere in the world of religious dedication to posit this as any fundamental human 'need'.

Thirdly, then, we may examine a suggestion deriving from Devereux (1979: 21). He talks of rhythmic activities in both dreams and waking life as symbolising coitus or sexual arousal. Included are walking and dancing, including trance-type head bobbing of the kind seen in the lower-order 'Swahili' *maulidi*. They are, as already mentioned, the male counterparts to the similarly trance-type body movements occurring among women at spirit possession dances. That is to say, the male Muslim use of the body in *maulidi* complements that of women in spirit possession, which is an activity condemned by Islamic clerics but nevertheless widespread among Muslim women and originating from and still practised among non-Muslims. It is, in fact, often explicitly sexual in its movements. Therefore, if Devereux's speculation is correct, men's dance and bodily movements are tacitly or, in his words, 'symbolically' sexual, while those of women possessed by spirits are consciously expressed as such.

We could go further on this line and suggest that Muslim men's sexuality is buried or repressed by their religiosity whereas that of their womenfolk is not. Among non-Muslims, women and men of all ages openly dance with each other at all rites of passage which are celebrated communally, and sexually expressive gestures and movements are the norm for both genders, especially at funerals. Among the Muslims, it is only at weddings that men and women may dance with each other, and even this is reserved generally for younger people.

Paradoxically, Muslim women have a reputation among non-Muslim men and women for sexual licentiousness, which in fact refers to the love-making skills which Muslim women are taught as they grow up. Moreover, among the lower-order 'Swahili' or 'Digo' at least, it has now become the custom, as a number of women and men declared, for the women to leave their husbands in the event of disagreement or boredom, with the result that separation and divorce rates are high. This is contrasted with the low rates among the non-Muslims, among whom the men claim to continue to exert control over their womenfolk.

Is it the case, therefore, that the propensity of so-called poorer or lower-order Swahili men to include trance, bodily movements, head bobbing and dancing in their *maulidi* is linked to their comparative lack of control over their women, or, to put it another way, to their more equal relationship with their women? Thus, while their womenfolk use the non-Muslim context of spirit possession, the men appear to choose the Muslim *maulidi* to express publicly their sexual distinctiveness. Given the higher value accorded to Islam by both men and women, the result is a hierarchy of male over female bodily expression.

The two explanations, the political and the supposedly ethno-psychoanalytic, need not in fact be incompatible. Indeed, I would suggest that the hierarchy of men over women in the Islamic religious sphere reflects a number of others: of 'Arab' over 'Swahili' *maulidi*; of high-status over lesser Muslims; and of Islamic beliefs and practices over non-Muslim ones.

The key question here is whether, as Devereux might be assumed to argue, bodily movement as symbolic of coitus is fundamental in this patterned expression of hierarchies. Or can we counter-argue that these social differences of rank and power find their expression in bodily movement as well as in other activities, and that the sexual innuendoes in such rhythmic movement are a possible but not inevitable aspect?

CONCLUSION

I end on this question of whether or how much these explanations of a mixed socio-political, interpersonal, gender and emotional nature are acceptable. The point is that there are still more explanations which could be given, but I will not extend the list further. None, however, is any other than speculative. Any human action can be attributed with an infinite number of meaningful associations. Dancing in dreams or waking life may well symbolise the rhythmic movements of coitus, a suggestion which, while remaining undemonstrable, is intuitively plausible. But, beyond this possibly universal feature, it is the relationship of the particular dance to other such dances and to the play of power relations between rich and poor, high and low status, allegedly pure and impure, and women and men, that provides the context in which people's imaginations work endlessly at interpretations, whether they are those of the outside analyst or those of the performers themselves. I suggest that this critical element of the play of power relations is the point at which ethnopsychoanalysis and anthropology meet.

BIBLIOGRAPHY

Deluz, A. (1979) 'George Devereux: a portrait', in R. H. Hook (ed.) *Fantasy and Symbol: Studies in Anthropological Interpretation*. London and New York: Academic Press.
Devereux, G. (1967) *From Anxiety to Method in the Behavioral Sciences*. The Hague and Paris: Mouton.
—— (1979) 'Fantasy and symbol as dimensions of reality', in R. H. Hook (ed.) *Fantasy and Symbol: Studies in Anthropological Interpretation*. London and New York: Academic Press.
Legendre, P. (1976) *Jouir du pouvoir*. Paris: Les Editions de Minuit.
Lévi-Strauss, C. (1979) 'Pythagoras in America', in R. H. Hook (ed.) *Fantasy and Symbol: Studies in Anthropological Interpretation*. London and New York: Academic Press.
Lienhardt, P. (1959) *Swifa: Medicine Man*. Oxford: Oxford University Press.
Moore, R. H. (1977) 'The Lamu Maulidi', unpublished paper presented to the Institute for African Studies, University of Nairobi.
Sagan, E. (1985) *At the Dawn of Tyranny*. London and Boston: Faber.

5 Trauma and ego-syntonic response
The Holocaust and 'The Newfoundland Young Yids', 1985

Nigel Rapport

This article follows the reaction by a number of Jewish friends to intimations made in Canada in the mid-1980s – and one Newfoundland newspaper article in particular – that the genocide of Jews in the Second World War (the Holocaust) was a hoax and part of an ongoing Jewish 'conspiracy'. It examines the social process whereby the friends organise themselves into a group so as to offer a joint response. This I do by focusing in detail on the interaction between them one evening shortly after the newspaper article appears. I offer the case-study as a comment on Devereux's notion of collective activities representing 'Ego-syntonic outlets'.

EGO-SYNTONISM

[B]oth organised and spontaneous social movements and processes are possible not because all individuals participating in them are identically (and sociologistically) motivated, but because a variety of authentically subjective motives may seek and find an Ego-syntonic outlet in the same type of collective activity. (Devereux 1978: 126)

Devereux distinguished between social or sociologistic mandates and motives, on the one hand, and subjective or psychological ones, on the other. These represented two domains, distinct 'universes of discourse', he argued, and it was absurd to attempt to reduce one to the other (1978: 133). Rather, in academic modelling, complementarity had to be recognised between them: they should be seen to 'fit together', 'through interplay and mutual reinforcement' (1978: 119); to be linked by 'something resembling feedback mechanisms' (1978:129). One significant feedback mechanism, for example, was the phenomenon of ego-syntonism, as outlined in the above quotation (also see Hook, 1979: 5): a process whereby a number of discrete consciousnesses became harmonically attuned to one another.

Methodologically, Devereux felt, the recognition of ego-syntonism was an advance in the explanation of the processes of sociation, of interaction and participation, because the collective act (the family meal, the clan ritual, the regional market, the national war) no longer needed to be construed in terms of either a homogeneous set of individual experiences or a single massive, social one. Instead, in the collective act 'society and culture' provided the medium, the channel, the occasion, for the public actualisation, ratification and gratification (in different ways and to different extents) of any number of individual meanings and motivations (1978: 127–8).

Certainly, the notion of ego-syntonism would appear a useful instrument in the continuing problematic of construing relations between 'the individual' and 'the collective', between the personal and the public (cf. Rapport, 1990). However, while mentioning the 1956 Hungarian uprising and weekly church-going as revolutionary and conservative exemplifications respectively, Devereux hardly described how precisely a variety of individual meanings and motivations did achieve collective embodiment. He spoke somewhat vaguely of 'differently motivated persons coming to perceive a given historical moment or event as suitable for a variety of gratifications' (1978: 128), but he hardly described such process in detail. This I attempt here. In particular, I focus on the negotiation of a particular code of interactional exchange. Through this, a set of young Jewish friends (who style themselves 'The Newfoundland Young Yids', or simply 'The Young Yids', or even 'The Y.Y.') establish definite boundaries around themselves, and respond to a newspaper article which has incited them by having a letter published in the same organ. It is by negotiating between them an agreed switch in behavioural code that the friends orchestrate a collective response; they come to agree, in short, upon the mandates of a collective Jewish trauma, while maintaining, none the less, distinct individual meanings of what Jewishness entails.

But let me not pre-empt my argument. First, I provide more background details of the case. Then I present an extended dramatic reconstruction of 'The Young Yids' in interaction; and finally I return to the implications of the case study for Devereuxian ego-syntonism.

THE ETHNOGRAPHIC SETTING

Newfoundland was England's earliest colony (1497); only in 1949 did it vote to become the tenth and newest part of Canada: 'The Happy Province'. Its population total is small, at approximately 580,000 (a density of less than 4 per square mile), and its economy remains 'underdeveloped'.[1] Thus Newfoundland retains the tag of Canada's 'Have-Not Province'.[2] Ninety-eight per cent of the population of Newfoundland is of Irish and English (West Country) extraction.[3] Only in the provincial capital of St John's (population 150,000) is this ethnic duality broadened, with a smattering of more recently arrived immigrants (and refugees): Vietnamese, Chinese, Greeks, Eastern Europeans, Pakistanis, Filipinos, American Indians and Jews (cf. Gilad, 1989).

The Newfoundland Jewish community is small, but economically quite established (see Kahn, 1987); from its St John's base, it services the island through retail and wholesale concerns such as clothing and hardware. Spurred by Eastern European pogroms, the first documented Jewish refugees reached Newfoundland in the 1890s. By 1909 St John's was host to sufficient for them officially to found The Hebrew Congregation of Newfoundland (although the first synagogue was not built until 1931). By 1921 the congregation totalled fourteen families, and by 1934, thirty-seven. The Second World War vitalised the community further (following a trough during the later Depression years) with an influx of Allied servicemen as well as European refugees; a second synagogue opened at the second city of Corner Brook. Since then, however, the Newfoundland congregation has declined, with its children progressing along a common immigrant path and transferring to the more lucrative Canadian mainland, and parents retiring near them (if not to Florida and California). By the 1980s there were only around twenty families, and it was becoming increasingly difficult to afford the upkeep of a *shul* (synagogue) and the living of a rabbi.

Occasionally, nevertheless, grown-up children do stay and work on the island. Moreover, in recent years these have been joined by a number of young Jewish adults from the mainland, who have come to finish their education at St John's university, or to teach there, or to get valuable experience in their profession (medicine or law, often) before returning to the more competitive mainland fray, or simply to experience a 'Third World country' and offer it their services. When I was conducting participant-observation fieldwork in St John's in 1984–5 (see Rapport, 1987, 1988), these young Jewish adults from the Canadian mainland, supplemented by one or two locals, formed something of a discrete set, speaking and meeting regularly. Their common Jewishness was the overt reason for their friendships, and the need to maintain Jewish identities in a gentile milieu. There was also the stated desire (since all were single) maybe, even here, to find a mate; in the meantime, they could provide a surrogate family for one another. True, they were invited into the homes of local Jewish families, but on many occasions it was together as a group that they celebrated Jewish holy days and ate kosher food in one another's rented rooms. Also together they started practising Israeli folk-dancing in the *shul* hall, learning Hebrew at the rabbi's house and travelling away to parties and conferences on the mainland to liaise with the umbrella

Maritime Confederation of Young Jewish Adults. And they started calling themselves 'The Newfoundland Young Yids'; it was a private name, a bit of a joke, but in its inversion of stigma it was also a statement of intent. For it was their wish to further the public status of Jewishness in an environment where the predominant religious expressions were Protestant and Catholic. But, more than this, they also hoped to claim an identity for themselves in contradistinction to the local old guard; as The Newfoundland Young Yids, they could represent their voices as those of young adults independent from the established Jewish community elders. Then, early in 1985, there was an incident which proved particularly opportune for a more public expression of these motivations.

The occasion was the appearance of the weekly *ned 'n' me* column in the widely read and respected local Newfoundland newspaper, *The Evening Telegram*. Dubbing itself 'The People's Paper', while flying the emblem of a Union Jack and boasting '1879 – Our 106th Year – 1984', the newspaper thus combined tradition and dependability with modernity and provincial independence. *ned 'n' me* was an idiosyncratic column written by the pseudonymous 'Mike Murphy', which, in the narrative idiom of a pub landlord having conversations with his regular ('ned') and not-so-regular customers, opined upon issues of the moment. In the edition in question (23 February), the column had touched upon the celebrated criminal trials of two mainland Canadians, Keegstra and Zundel. Both were later convicted, but at the time Zundel was defending himself from prosecution for disseminating a pamphlet entitled *The Hoax of the Twentieth Century* which described the extermination of six million Jews between 1939 and 1945 as propaganda and lies, while Keegstra was fighting prosecution for teaching schoolchildren in his classroom that behind two thousand years of ills in Christian society lay a Jewish conspiracy. Let me quote from the article, which 'Mike Murphy' entitles 'Freedom (?) of speech'.[4] Here, the pub landlord narrates how one night a new, strangely frightened customer took him to task for naïveté:

'This is a free country.'
'The hell it is,' he said. 'Ask Keegstra. Ask Zundel.'
'Who?'
'You see!' he said. 'You're like most Canadians. You don't know that Keegstra and Zundel are being prosecuted by the courts for reading what they want to read, making up their own minds about the truth of what the books have to say and, then, expressing an opinion publicly.'
'That's ridiculous,' I said. 'A Canadian is free to say what he likes.'
'Ha!' he snorted. 'Maybe that was true when you Newfies joined Canada. It's not that way today. . . .'

'I can't believe that,' I said. 'Things like that can't happen here.'
'That's what the Germans thought until Hitler proved them wrong,' he said. '. . . I was a high school teacher in Medicine Hat, in charge of the school library. I ordered from the States, a dozen copies of a book called *The Hoax of the Twentieth Century*, and since it is one of the 1,200 banned books, the Canadian Customs confiscated them. So I smuggled a few copies in, by way of a travelling friend. The SIS [Canadian Secret Police] found out and I've been on the run ever since.'
'And they have orders to liquidate you,' I said. . . .
'Oh, I think the orders came from outside the SIS,' he said. 'Sort of like their taking a "contract to kill" on me.'
'What?' I said. 'You are crazy, you know? Who would get the SIS to kill you?'
'I suppose,' he said, 'someone who doesn't want me to read and talk about *The Hoax of the Twentieth Century*.'
I couldn't believe my ears, but By Golly, he could be right. That kind of thing happens to the dictatorships. Why not in Canada? . . .
'Well, come in tomorrow,' I said, 'and we'll have another drink and a chat.'
'Me?' he said. 'No. I'm getting murdered in the morning.'

Shortly after the weekend edition with the above column appeared, the phone lines between the young Jewish friends were buzzing. The others agreed with a suggestion of Izzy's that 'something had to be done'. Hence, a 'business meeting' of 'The Y.Y.' was called for the following (Sunday) evening, with Pnina's apartment as the venue. Before I introduce more (fictionalised) names, however, and describe their interaction, let me explain a little more of my intent.

The friends did not usually call their get-togethers 'business meetings'. Indeed, this usage left them slightly embarrassed and the designation would be followed by a chuckle. What is significant is how commensurate 'business meeting' was with the rhetoric of this particular interaction as a whole. Not only did the young Jews meet to conduct adult business, then, but, as we shall see, they also sought a more public, institutional name for themselves. Furthermore, they adopted, *ad hoc*, a formal agenda, a chairman and a secretary keeping 'minutes'. Here was a distinct behavioural code, a code such as may have befitted a committee or council, and which I shall term a conciliar rhetoric.

By instituting a conciliar rhetoric as a frame for their interaction, the friends achieved a number of things. First, as mentioned, by proclaiming themselves 'Newfoundland Young Yids', they inverted a felt stigma and claimed identities of which they were determined to feel confident and proud. But then by uniting publicly behind an institutional name and an impersonal way of speaking they also distanced their pronouncements from their individual, everyday lives and selves. Thus they made public statements which were not necessarily 'theirs', and concerning an issue (anti-semitism) and an event (the Holocaust) which did not necessarily concern them.

In the following scene, then, the friends switch in and out of the formal behaviours and linguistic formulae of a conciliar rhetoric as they decide how to respond to the incitement and prejudice they see in 'Mike Murphy's' article; they formalise and defend the boundaries of their Jewish group against this and other gentile pejoration, but at the same time maintain routine individual identities (Jewish and other) which are fed by other meanings and motivations. I hope to show these individuals, by intermittently coming together within this collective rhetorical framework, addressing their enemies as a legitimate and effective religious group, using a language of adult, public debate and steeped in the security of the propriety which such debating entails, while also distancing their 'private' individual selves from the historical trauma of which their public voices declare themselves to be direct descendants.

And so to Pnina's apartment. *Pnina Gould* is a dietician at the University Medical Center. In her late twenties, she was born in Ottawa and has lived in St John's for three years. The first to arrive for their meeting is *Izzy (Israel) Horovitz*. Izzy, in his mid-twenties, is a civil servant in the provincial government's Department of Energy, Mines and Resources. He was born in Newfoundland but feels ambivalent about calling it 'home'. As a teenager he lived for a couple of years in Israel – The *Aretz*, The Land – and now that he is back he still likes to pepper his talk with Hebrew and Yiddish words; for him, asking a bemused waiter for 'the *cheshbon*' instead of 'the bill', surrounded by a group of laughing Jewish friends from the mainland to whom he can act as something of a host – this, alone, feels like real belonging.

Next to arrive is *Basil LaRusic*. A teacher of social science, in his late twenties, Basil was born in Cardiff (Wales) and has lived in St John's for a year. Finally, arriving together are *Mirium Hagentasch* and *Dina Schwartz* with a message that *Rachel Fernstein* will be a little late. Mirium is an occupational therapist at The Sisters of the Beatitudes General Hospital; in her early thirties, she was born in Montreal but has lived in St John's for almost seven years. Dina, in her mid-twenties, was born in Halifax and has lived here for two years while reading for an MA in folklore at the university. Rachel, also mid-twenties, works as an adviser in community health; she was born in Toronto but has been in St John's for three years.

Here is the interaction which I recorded between the above in my field journal that evening – assisted by the notes I was able to take at the time in my role as the minute-keeper, and my identity (in this account) as 'Basil LaRusic'.

THE INTERACTION

A pine table is appetisingly decorated with opened bottles of wine and the remains of various savoury dips. Izzy and Mirium are slouched on a leather sofa, while Basil has pulled out a chair from the dining table, and Pnina and Dina are propped up on large scatter cushions on the floor.

'Anyway, you guys, shall we start the meeting,' Izzy says, cleaning his fingers on his handkerchief, 'seeing Rachel's gonna be late? Here, I wrote out a sort of agenda.' He pulls out a piece of paper from his pocket, unfolds it and reads, 'Item Number One: The chairman of the Maritime Jewish Confederation called me to say he wants to come over from Halifax next month and give us a talk, okay? If we tell him what on.'

There are murmurs of interest.

'Second Item: We need to settle on a proper name for our group and kind'a schematise our goals. Like, a first thing, and Item Three on the agenda, is that we need to write a reply to that *ned 'n' me* article yesterday on Keegstra and Zundel.'

'God, that was disgusting! Did you see that Dina?'

'Hey, hold on, Pnina. First things first, okay? So, lastly, Item Four on the agenda is we should set a date for Rachel to tell us about that conference she went to on Soviet Jewry.' Izzy stops reading and looks satisfied. 'Oh, Bas, will you take minutes?'

'What! Why me? Anyhow, I haven't got a pen.'

'Why can't you, Izzy?'

'Because I'm the chairman, Dina, and I'll be speaking.'

Pnina laughs, but finds Basil pen and paper. 'So fire away, Mr Chairperson.'

'God,' Basil moans. 'Why do I feel like in Russia?'

'Oh, come on,' Mirium laughs, 'someone ought to. Right. Before we can schematise our group goals, I think we should define our problems.'

'No, surely we ought to kind'a brief our goals and objectives before we get to problems, eh? And I think our first goal should be Outreach.'

'Right, Pnina! Got that Bas?' Basil nods and writes as Izzy and the others hum agreement: they need to reach other young Jews in Newfoundland and tell them about their group and its activities. 'What about all these Jews at the university I keep hearing about?' Izzy continues. 'Can't we get them to sort of come out of the closet? Motivate them to come, and all this. What about some posters around the Medical Center, Pnina?'

'Or an information table like Christian Fellowship puts up in the Students' Union!' Pnina laughs. 'No. I doubt it'd work, frankly. I mean a high profile's fine but I'm not sure there's really the source to tap, eh? I don't think the Jews there'd wanna be attracted.'

'Right,' Dina nods, 'same in folklore. I mean there's professors like Paul Cohen, and in sociology there's Jake Hornung – '

'Hornung! Hey, he's not from Corner Brook, is he?' Izzy enthuses. ''Cos there are about thirty Jews out in west Newfoundland and "Hornung" kind'a rings a bell. That's where the Levys were from. You know, "Levy's Jeans" in the mall. But they got ostracised for being Jewish and had to live outside the community. And now they aren't really Jewish any more.'

'Sorry. Jake Hornung's Californian, Izzy! But, anyway, I don't think they're really into Judaism.'

'But why not? Aren't they interested in their identities?' Izzy sounds resentful. 'Hey! That reminds me. There's a new Jew in town, guys! Mark Coser's his name. A doctor, I heard.'

'Is that right?' Mirium exclaims, jokily over-exaggerating her interest and 'availability'. 'Tell me more!'

'I'll try and get him to come along to the next Israeli dancing,' Izzy promises. 'Nice young doctor for you little ladies.'

'God! We've become such awful *yentes* since coming here. Gossiping about everyone,' Pnina bemoans. 'And right after the day God's been listening too! Isn't it a sin.'

'Yis, Boy. It's some sin, wha'?' Dina provides the Newfoundland brogue. 'A sin against Lard T'undering Jaysus too, Boy, to be sure.' The rest laugh. 'Oh I must tell you: I went to see my doctor last week and he thought I was a Newfie! It was so funny. He told me to eat less fat and stay off the fish-and-brews for a spell.' All are amused at the idea of them eating the local speciality of salt cod and ship's biscuit fried in lard. 'I nearly died!'

'But I find most people here don't know what a Jew is,' Mirium says and the others hum sympathetically. 'I tell some of my patients and they think it means I'm American or something!'

'Right,' Izzy agrees. 'Buddy at work wouldn't believe I didn't believe in Jesus and didn't celebrate Christmas and stuff, or even have a Christmas tree at home: "If Catholics and Protestants can *both* have one", he said, "how come Jews can't?"' They laugh. 'He said how the Christian Brothers taught him only Christians got proper ethics and know how to behave and be charitable and all this. Anyway, you guys, let's get back to the agenda. We gotta get a proper name for the group so anyone who wants to can get in touch.'

'What about putting our name and a phone number under "Religious Organisations" in the *Yellow Pages*?'

'Good idea, Dina. And we could run an ad in the *Telegram*: "Anyone Like A Kosher Friday Night Meal?" '

'Right, Mirium. Or we could write an article for the student newspaper 'cos they have a section for community news. Free, I think, too.'

'Free! Free! *Chinam! Chinam!*' Pnina jumps in with one of Izzy's favourite Hebrew words, before he has a chance to, and the others laugh.

Just then, there is a knock on the door and Rachel walks in: 'Hi, gang! Sorry I'm so late. I'm working for this health educator at the moment who's worse than the Bitch of Buchenwald – excuse my French.' Rachel hangs her coat over a chair as greetings are exchanged, and then sits on a scatter cushion: 'So what have I missed, guys?'

'Bas. Tell her the minutes so far. You sure been scribbling some.'

'Right, Izzy. Well, first, Mirium said we should schematise our problems before we set out our goals. Then Pnina said we ought to brief our objectives in order to define our problems . . .'

Mirium and then Pnina and the others blush and laugh as Basil reads back the highfalutin' report.

'Oh my, Basil!' Izzy cackles. 'You're something else writing all that down! You're too much!'

Rachel, however, is not sidetracked, and after each point she responds with a serious 'Definitely'. Then when Basil finishes she adds: 'Am *I* down there, yet?'

'You know, looking back this has been a very good year for the group, hasn't it, guys?' Dina suggests.

'It's been the *only* year!'

'Yeah, okay, Mirium. But I mean we began as separate people, then we got together and held our first meeting of The Y.Y.s, remember? Then we diversified into all kinds of things: Hebrew lessons, Israeli dancing, Soviet Jewry – Night-clubbing on Saturday night!' They laugh. 'Hey, you know what? We should write a report, a kind of diary of our activities. And then we could send it to Hannah and Debbie, and anyone else who leaves.'

'The alumni!' Basil jokes.

'Hey, that reminds me. I think Soviet Jewry should be written down as one of our group goals. Definitely.'

'But isn't that already taken care of in "Outreach", Rachel?' Mirium ponders.

'So tell us about Toronto and the Soviet Jewry conference, Rachel,' Pnina asks.

'Of course! We haven't seen you since,' Mirium is reminded.

'Great, really! It really fired me up. 'Cos it was all about how Judaism's something you gotta work at, not just something you're born into and that's it. So in Russia, they don't allow it. And in New York these days you'll likely see a Black guy explaining *gefilte* fish to a Chinaman! So it's not just ethnicity, any more,' Rachel explains and the others laugh at her example. 'Anyhow, they said we should arrange something special for Human Rights Day on December 10; and then we should light candles for Soviet refuseniks in *shul*, and leave a special seat vacant for them as well, to signify.'

'We could leave 'em three in ours!' Dina jokes. 'A row even!'

'Okay. But joking aside, they said communities all across Canada should organise some public reminder of the dissidents' plight.'

'Hey look, you guys, couldn't we set a special date for this Soviet Jewry stuff. We got other things to discuss tonight. Let's get back to the agenda. So my little buddy in Halifax, Mr Harvey Greenspan, informs me that the chairman of The Maritime Jewish Confederation's gonna be here one night and wants to give us a talk; if we had a subject. A chat more than a lecture he said: he's only a young feller himself. Got a Ph.D. But nice guy. So what on?'

'How about what makes us Jews what we are?' Rachel suggests, and there are murmurs of approval.

'Is this talk gonna be for members only, like, or can I bring some friends from work?'

'Let's keep it members only, Mirium. You can't say things properly otherwise.'

'Or how about a talk on something the rest of the community might like to come to as well? Like a history of Jewish settlement in Atlantic Canada.'

'That's a good idea, Pnina,' Mirium agrees. 'And wouldn't that be something your parents'd come to as well, Izzy? . . . They immigrated here from Russia, didn't they?'

'Well, Dad says how he doesn't rightly know where they came from 'cos the country changed hands so often. First it was Lithuania, then Poland, then Germany, then Russia! Then after Auschwitz he went to Italy, and then finally came here 'cos Israel was out of bounds. So he made his first buck and he's been here ever since! And I think he'd be scared to leave now. He's like the rabbi, eh. He thinks all the world just wants the Jews dead.'

'I guess you can't really blame him!'

'Right, Mirium! Really,' Rachel agrees.

'I don't know though. I wouldn't wanna agree with much of what the rabbi thinks,' Dina shakes her head. 'Remember that sermon he gave about the Holocaust, in the Memorial Service? "God willed the Holocaust and it is just part of some bigger logic which we can't fathom. Or not yet, anyway, 'cos it's still too close for us to see it in focus." Now, is that thinking weird, Boy, or wha'?'

'Well. The rabbi knows the rules, after all, Girl.'

'Yeah, but Izzy, remember how after they televised our Holocaust Memorial Evening all these people round St John's called up the rabbi and Gaby and said they couldn't understand anti-semitism, and went on quoting the Bible against it?'

'Right, Mirium. I mean generally this is such a sane country. It's not like some places where you sort of feel violence under the surface all the time. Israel, for example! I mean, don't let's get paranoid, now.'

'I don't think it's paranoid, Dina. You know they painted swastikas and "Death to the Jews" on the *shul* a few years back.'

'Yeah, but come on. That's really unusual for round here, Izzy,' Pnina claims.

'Okay, so what about this *ned 'n' me* article? Don't you think that's frightening and something we gotta do something about. Like I put on the agenda?'

'Sure, Izzy. That's lunatic. All about some Jewish conspiracy, eh? I mean, it's a joke!' Dina laughs.

'We gotta do something, though,' Pnina agrees. 'It's plain ignorant. Crazy!'

'Parochial claptrap,' Basil says.

'Right,' Mirium nods. 'I mean on the one hand you wanna say, "who's gonna believe this trash, eh?" But then this kind'a thing can incite people too.'

'Look, people. This is pure hate literature and lies, and there are laws against it in the Criminal Code,' Rachel states. 'So I vote we write to the *Telegram* and say what "Mr so-called Murphy"'s doing's illegal. And if he does it again he could be prosecuted.'

'Yeah. That'd show 'em up,' Pnina agrees.

'Okay, so look. How about if Izzy and I draft a letter to the *Telegram* and bring it along to Israeli dancing on Wednesday. Then we can all see what we think before we send it, right?' Rachel looks around and the others nod consent.

'Good idea,' Mirium adds.

'Right. But we gotta do it soon. That's why I thought we should all meet tonight. I think the rabbi's phoned the editor already and complained.'

'How are we gonna sign it? With our names?'

'No. I think it should be from the group, Mirium,' Rachel counters.

'But hold on, you guys. We don't even have a name for ourselves, yet!' Izzy complains.

'How about "The Jewish Council"?' Rachel wonders.

'"The Jewish Directorate General"!' Basil sounds sarcastic.

'Why not simply "Concerned Jews". Or "The Jewish Community"?'

'No I don't think Gaby would like that, Mirium. That's what he puts when he writes stuff as president of the *shul*. Anyway, I think we should make our own statement, you know, as a group.'

'How about simply "The Group". Or *Ha'Kvutsa*, since we're meant to be Hebrews.'

'Oh come on, Pnina. Half the people *here* wouldn't know what that meant.'

'Okay, smarty-pants. So you think up something, Izzy. Uh, how about "The Israel Group"?'

'No. I don't want my name being used.'

'"*Shalom*"?'

'No. Sounds like a Peace Group.'

'Well I give up, Izzy. What other words can you think of that people associate immediately with Jews? "Jerusalem"?'

'Why not just "The Young Yids"?' Dina jokes and the others laugh.

'"The Council for Soviet Jewry Action".' Rachel motions the title in lights, and grins. 'Anyway, look guys, Izzy and I'll sort something out and then we can all finalise things on Wednesday. Okay?'

'Hey. Have you been watching Zundel on the News? Marching in and out of court, with his cronies in those steel helmets! Scary stuff, eh?' Pnina shivers.

'Yeah! Really,' Dina shakes her head in disbelief.

'And God: those lawyers! Telling Auschwitz survivors how they can't be sure anyone was gassed.' Mirium tuts.

'Well. Like my dad always says: "*Schwer a Yid zu sei*".'

'What's that, Izzy?' Pnina jumps up excitedly.

'"It's hard to be a Jew": "*Schwer a Yid zu sei*". Yes, Boy!'

'"*Schwer a Yid . . .*"'

'"*Zu sei*".'

'"*Zu sei*", "*Schwer a Yid zu sei*", "*Schwer a Yid zu sei*",' Pnina repeats to herself. 'That's great. I'll remember that. "*Oy! Schwer a Yid zu sei*".' She giggles.

'Well, as chairman of this meeting, how about if we close things up for now? I'm starving already. Anyone else wanna join me for some fish 'n' chips at Murphy's Cafe?' Izzy's idea meets with approval. 'Write up them minutes, Bas, and I'll send 'em off to Halifax,' he adds and they start clearing things away into the kitchen.

Over the next couple of days, numerous phone-calls pass between them as Rachel and Izzy compose a letter. The wording is finally agreed upon at Wednesday's session of Israeli dancing and the letter dispatched. And, on 2 March, the next Saturday, the following appears in *The Evening Telegram* print:

Sir,

Upon reading your *ned 'n' me* article last Saturday we were left with the impression that journalistic freedom (?) had been taken a step too far.

Freedom of speech is important in any democracy and we're in big trouble without it. . . . [However], we do not support, as the *Telegram* must and has, freedom to tell lies. We do not believe a person should be free to disseminate racism and the literature of hate. The Keegstra and Zundel prosecutions are not, as Mr. 'Murphy' so naively put it in his column, due to their mere expression of an opinion in public. The prosecution of Zundel relates to Section 117 of the Canadian Criminal Code – the 'spreading of false information that caused or is likely to cause social and racial intolerance'. The prosecution of Keegstra relates to Section 281-2 of the Criminal Code – 'wilfully promoting hatred against an identifiable group'.

Freedom of the press should be considered a responsibility as well as a right. While anyone – including Mr. 'Murphy' – is entitled to express his/her views in private, it is inexcusable for a responsible newspaper to publish an article which suggests the Keegstra and Zundel prosecutions to be unjust. Sections of the Canadian Criminal Code were written for the Zundels and Keegstras of the world. We suggest you read it!

The Soviet Jewry Action Council, St John's

THE INTERACTION ANALYSED

A council, according to Richards (1971: 1–2), may be defined as an institutional grouping of people which meets in a regular place and with some consistency over time, in order to reach joint decisions; its institutionality entails membership being limited, and situated proceedings, verbal and other, being conventionalised. In Devereuxian terms, a council represents a collective activity imbued with social mandates and motives.

What especially interests me here, in relation to the case I have been outlining, is the language involved. Richards describes council language as 'conventional'. Borrowing from Bernstein, we might be more precise in defining it as 'public language'. This Bernstein describes as highly structured, even ritualised, communication (phraseology, sequencing, intonation), which best bespeaks routine, order, role and social-structural status quo between a specified set of people (1964: *passim*). Indeed, the restrictiveness of public language fosters in its usage a certain social solidarity, emphasising the collective identity of an 'us' over the individual elaborations of various 'me's. Thus, its restrictions signal to members and outsiders alike the normative practices and arrangements of a group: commonality, shared expectations and loyalty to symbolic convention (1972: 476).[5]

Bernstein then goes on to tie the practice of public language primarily to a particular social group: the English working class. But this seems to me an unnecessary impoverishment. As Paine rightly argues (1976: 74), we should rather expect public language to be a resource which different people might use in different situations as interactions assume different priorities; a strategy for problem solving in particular social contexts (Gal, 1989: 351–2). Similarly, Richards envisages that, institutionality notwithstanding, conciliar patterns of interaction could also be adopted by informally constituted groups which happen to have recourse to a set of procedural rules (1971: 2–3). Here, then, is a mode of proceeding and speaking, 'conciliar rhetoric' if you will, which individuals might adopt for the situational purpose of constituting a group: establishing identity, expressing commonality, fostering belonging; fusing individual speakers and listeners.

Moreover, it is in terms of such conciliar rhetoric that the above scene gives clues to a process whereby individual Jewishness could be said to amount to collective Jewish trauma, and meet in ego-syntonic response. For here was an exchange which was structured by the *ad hoc* adoption of a formal conciliar procedure and imbued with a certain restricted intonation, which eventuated in the coming together of a number of Jewish friends and their meeting in a collective statement.

Let me elaborate. 'The Soviet Jewry Action Council, St John's' is a title which the friends had not used to describe their association hitherto. The title was resorted to precisely to deal with the problem of the *ned 'n' me* article. Similarly, as I mentioned, the friends rarely referred to their get-togethers as 'business meetings' and never with the seriousness they managed to muster in their use of it on this occasion. The same goes for the set of titular and technical terms, and their attempted solemn intonation, which peppered the talk: 'Mr Chairperson', 'Chairman', 'minute-taker', 'item', 'agenda', 'seminar', 'schematising goals', 'briefing objectives', 'outreach', 'The Maritime Jewish Confederation', 'Mr Harvey Greenspan', and so on. Here was a far more formal, abstract and impersonal verbal array than usually characterised their interactions. Furthermore, besides the words, the procedure of following an agenda provided a behavioural convention which framed the whole meeting: the kind of attitude they expected of themselves, the type of matters discussed, the nature of the conclusions to be reached.

More exactly, then, what was it that these individuals *did* collectively affirm through their conciliar proceedings? Firstly, that they were a group. They began as 'separate people', as Dina significantly phrased it, then they 'got together and held meetings'; they institutionalised themselves. Now, they held 'business meetings', business being the newcomer's route to possession and belonging (as it was for Izzy's father who stayed put, having made his first buck). Moreover, like all serious business institutions, they had also 'diversified', investing in different enterprises such as Hebrew lessons and Israeli dancing. Similarly, they had group strategies and business targets: they placed the serious business on the agenda (*ned 'n' me*) as the third item, when discussion would be in full swing, and even then they ended up dealing with it (and Keegstra and Zundel) at the very end; also, they planned media events and recruitment drives, and discussed which informations to publicise and publish where (in the alumni newsletter, for instance, as opposed to the letter to the *Telegram*). But they were not merely a business institution, they were also a family one: they cooked and ate together, they touched, laughed and quarrelled, they allowed for the foibles – the pique, the self-advertisement – of fellow-members; they forwent sexual relations for more inclusive sibling-like ones. The business and the family identities combined, perhaps, as the group's outside and inside faces respectively: to the outside they were The Soviet Jewry Action Council, while inside they remained the familiar 'Y.Y.'. In fine, now they were a group as institutional as others they could name, from Newfoundland-based ones to Canada-wide; and even if small and new, they expected to occupy their rightful group place beside these others, for example in the Yellow Pages telephone directory of local religious organisations.

Secondly, the adultness of their group was asserted. For here they were working alongside the rabbi, the president of the *shul* (Gaby) and the wider Newfoundland Jewish community, co-ordinating their activities and yet making separate statements. Moreover, this was an inherently Jewish adultness, serious in its commitment both to a continuing appreciation of the trauma of the past, the prejudices of the present, and the dangers of the future. Hence they added their voice to local Holocaust Memorial Services, to reminders about the ongoing violation of Jewish cultural rights, and to calls for a constructive ethnicity.

Thirdly, the normality of their Jewish identity in Newfoundland was averred. Newfoundland may represent a religiously dualistic, historically ignorant environment but they were prepared to break the mould: to say that, among other ethnicities, there were Newfies, there were also Chinese and Blacks, and there were Jews. These had to be treated openly, without discrimination; also without shame, for Jewishness was not something to hide in the closet. Therefore, their group would work on Outreach, on familiarity with Yiddish Hebrew ('*yente*', '*Chinam*'), on advertising Jewish customs and forums in the local press ('Friday night meals', 'community news').

In sum, partaking of conciliar proceedings, these individuals took part in a social process of group formation, and instituted a common boundary around themselves. In particular, through their interaction they protected themselves from a Jewish trauma, distanced themselves from it, while at the same time forming a solidary front because of it. Whatever it meant to them as individuals, if anything, beforehand, their public language led them to a defining of Jewish trauma as collective: as something pertaining to their common identity as members of a group even if not inherent in them as separate individuals.

But let me explain this latter point more fully. I have argued that the appearance of the *ned 'n' me* article (and the past and concurrent experiences and events with which it could be linked) was seen as traumatic. Here was the prime motivation behind these individuals engaging in group institutionalisation as well as the major mandate for their group action. Furthermore, the extent to which this trauma could be exorcised and kept distant provided a measure of group success. In short, here was a common Jewish trauma which was very much part-and-parcel of the group's identity and *raison d'être*, for it was in this trauma that the individual friends met. Thus, the construction of trauma, of violent implications in *ned 'n' me* and a wider anti-semitic ambience (swastikas, myopic Christian Brothers, *Schwer a Yid zu sei*), was as much part of the above scene as the solidifying of a united group against it: here was trauma as social need. Thus, the trauma I have spoken of so far may be described as a collective one and belonging to what Devereux denoted as the social or sociologistic domain.

In contradistinction to this, however, the meanings and motivations in what Devereux termed the subjective or psychologistic domain (which the social exchange of conciliar rhetoric served ego-syntonically to attune) might be expected to be quite distinct, if not diverse (cf. Rapport, 1986). This is evidenced, I suggest, in a number of ambivalences in the scene, of separations between individual and collective proceedings, of idiosyncrasies of attitude and expression. More specifically, there were ambivalences expressed, firstly, about conciliar rhetoric; then, about the aims of the group and its Jewish problems; lastly, about the robustness of the group and its potential for success.

To elaborate a little on these and the individuals particularly concerned, it was Izzy who introduced the conciliar rhetoric and he who remained most enamoured of it. For the others to accept it was, to some extent, also to accept a formal group of which Izzy proclaimed himself leader. It was true that, to them, Izzy was the native, the token Newfoundlander. However, this the others recognised as both an advantage and a disadvantage. He had better-established links with the native Jewish community, with the rabbi and Gaby, with the Maritime Jewish Confederation, but then his horizons were also narrower, his accent more parochial, his outlook more Newfie. It was clear to all, Izzy included, that he had not learnt to 'pass' as non-Jewish in professional circles, nor how to feel at home as a transient; he resented always standing out in Newfoundland. Hence, while the others allowed themselves to be co-opted by Izzy into the conciliar rhetoric of his group at some moments, at others they switched into more informal and personal language. Thus, Pnina teased Izzy about his 'chairmanship'; she and Mirium laughed in embarrassment at having their highfalutin' words reviewed, while Basil likened conciliar practice and the cavalier fashion in which Izzy had attempted to introduce it to the very totalitarianism they were there to combat. Always it was Izzy who called speakers back to the agenda, and particularly at those moments when their solidarity as a New-foundland Jewish group seemed most at risk: when the inexorable dualism of local religiosity was being aired, for example; when his use of Hebrew words was parodied; when a division between Canada and Israel was envisaged. Despite these efforts of Izzy's, moreover, few items on the agenda were ever resolved – a name for the group, for instance; its 'goals', 'objectives' and 'problems'; further dates for a meeting on Soviet Jewry or a talk by the Maritime Confederation chairman; and so on – while his attempts otherwise to quash informality were often simply ignored.

Besides Izzy, it was Rachel who most favoured conciliar rhetoric, using it from the outset as a point of contact with the group and a means of registering and recording belonging; thus, she was not happy until she appeared in the amber of the minutes and her earlier non-presence had been negated. But then it was also Rachel who was most 'fired up' about the external (Soviet) threat; and Rachel who, with Izzy, was probably the most uncertain about her individual adult identity at work (with the Bitch of Buchenwald). In short, Rachel and Izzy felt most comfortable within the conventional forms of public language. For the others it was a useful tool in external relations (letters, posters, adverts and so on), where anonymity and officiality imparted imposing strengths, and individuality needed pro-tection, but they rather lost patience when its restrictiveness threatened internal banter, flexibility and fun. It was natural enough that Rachel and Izzy should be most keen to compose the letter of riposte to the *Telegram*, finding in each other symbolic mates (even if not sexual ones).

Ambivalence about the aims of the group and its Jewish problems was expressed perhaps most by Dina and Mirium. Both felt rooted in a Canadian identity whose ethos contrasted sharply with an Israeli one stirred by violent undercurrents. Moreover, Mirium did not feel St John's was an anti-semitic environment at all, while Dina found the rabbi's philosophical interpretation of divinely inspired discrimination risible. Finally, when it came to the question of Jewish separatism, Pnina too distanced herself from Izzy's stereotypical views ('the world wants the Jews dead', 'Death to the Jews').

Probably it was Dina again who expressed most ambivalence about the robustness of the group and its potential for success. Just as the Newfound-land community was heading for the mainland and leaving whole rows empty in their old *shul*, and just as her professors elected an academic identity over a Jewish one, so she did not have much hope in their attracting more members. Pnina, moreover, had to agree: beyond themselves, there was little source to tap.

The picture which emerges from the scene, then, is very much of two elements, two domains. For here were individual meanings and motivations and here were group ones. Groupness manifested itself in a certain conciliar rhetoric. However, this was introduced and carried forward by, associated with, some individuals rather than others; groupness was allied more with some members' interests than others. A compromise, perhaps, was reached in the notion of 'The Y.Y. Group': however they were seen and named by the outside, it was as 'The Y.Y.' that, on the inside, they would know themselves. Here was an official title but it was private, it jokingly embraced the stigma, and it was less officious than 'The Soviet Jewry Action Council': here was a more personal version of conciliar rhetoric for internal consumption. Even so, within the compromise, the ambivalences and idiosyncrasies remained; individuals were more and less separate from the group, were members of 'The Y.Y.' in different ways and to different extents. Rachel had her campaigning zeal and political causes; Izzy had his manifesting of Newfoundland Judaism; Dina had her practising of Jewish 'folklore', its philosophy and physical activity; Pnina had her learning of Hebrew language and cooking; Mirium had her earnest searching for a Jewish mate; Basil had his marrying of anthropological research with an entertaining social life. None the less, these individuals *did* manage to come together, as in the above conversation, and agree: that they felt distant from Newfoundland culture; that the environment was narrow and exclusionary; that they wanted to meet and socialise with other Jews. Above all, they came together in finding the national television coverage of the Zundel trial and the *ned 'n' me* article, its Newfoundland corollary, traumatic; that is, 'lunatic' (Dina), 'ignorant' (Pnina), 'inciteful' (Mirium), 'parochial' (Basil), 'illegal' (Rachel) and 'frightening' (Izzy).

Bailey (1965: 9–15) has suggested that differentiation be made between councils which reach decisions by majority vote and those which prefer consensus. Examples of the latter may be found, he continues, where there is overriding concern with external relations, such as opposition to foreign bodies; for, then, consensus promotes the image of unanimity (and anonymity) within the group, however much a facade. Indeed, Kuper concurs (1971: 23), the maximising of a display of unanimity and a closing of ranks may be the council's primary intention, while any other decisions taken may be more *pro forma* than practical. Certainly here, consensus and a maximisation of the appearance of unanimity, solidarity and organisation were the primary group motivations, and the Soviet Jewry Action Council was a formalisation of relations in opposition to what were seen as hostile aspects of external gentile society.

However, there *was* a decision to write a letter and this did issue forth, even if it was produced outside the formal context of the council meeting. In conclusion, then, let us look at this consequence.

THE OUTCOME

In the same weekend edition of *The Evening Telegram* in which the letter from 'The Soviet Jewry Action Council' was printed, there also appeared the next *ned 'n' me* article (on a wholly different issue) and an editorial column entitled 'Ned 'n' Me'. And in the latter was to be found (in part) the following: .

> Would *The Evening Telegram* publish an article which had as its main and only purpose the arousing of hatred against a particular religious or racial group?
>
> The answer is a resounding No.
>
> Further, *The Evening Telegram* has never published such an article. . . .
>
> Rabbi [Uzi Fine] of St. John's maintains that a *Ned 'n' Me* column published Feb.23 in *The Evening Telegram* Saturday, Feb 23, was a thinly-veiled defence of anti-Semites and anti-Semitism.
>
> We have no wish to belittle or denigrate the concerns of Rabbi [Fine] or the other six people who expressed their concerns about the column, either by letter or by telephone. . . .
>
> We confess to being taken aback by the accusation that the article is anti-semitic. . . .
>
> Those objecting to the meaning of the column have placed their own definition on what was intended. That is not fair, and in our mind, it is not a true definition.
>
> Those who disagree with the column have the right and privilege of disagreeing; we defend and agree with that right and that privilege by publishing all of their statements.
>
> Important questions have been raised in this province and in this country recently about such fundamental issues as freedom of speech and the freedom to hold opinions and communicate them.
>
> Those questions are not answered by denying that they are legitimate questions and insisting that they not be asked. . . .

Paine has argued that the public languages of different groups may be seen to abut against one another; hence, while expressing solidarity between members of one group, the rhetorics metacommunicate disjunctions between groups (1976: 79). It is this which, I suggest, we can see happening here. In response to the letter from 'The Soviet Jewry Action Council', and the phone-call from the rabbi and a number of other communiqués, *The Evening Telegram* offers its own array of formal and abstract verbiage, parades its own flags and borders.

Nevertheless, to this extent, Izzy and Rachel and Pnina and Mirium and Dina and Basil do succeed. For they have formalised their internal relations as Newfoundland Young Yids, presented themselves as The Soviet Jewry Action Council to the outside world and had their position publicly recognised, even legitimised by a published response. There may be *The Evening Telegram* (the *Telegram*), Christian Fellowship, The Maritime Jewish Confederation and so on, but now there is also The Soviet Jewry Action Council ('The Y.Y.'), with its meetings, issues, lobbying and its possible turnover in membership. In Bailey's terms (1965: 10), the vertical cleavages dividing the friends as a group from others and structuring relations between them have become more clearly defined and expectable. 'The Young Yids' and their Jewishness have entered into an established arena of adult, open debate.

SUMMARY

The friends could not publicly call themselves 'The Israel Group', we heard from Izzy, because he did not want his name being used. Beneath the extreme self-centredness of this remark (or, perhaps, the excessive provincialism which Izzy associates with and expects from a Newfoundland milieu) is a neat encapsulation of the distinction Devereux would have us draw between collective and individual, between distinct but complementary social and psychological domains. The social, he would argue, provides an ego-syntonic outlet for the psychological: the singular social process or collective act composed of diverse individual meanings and psychological motivations. It is the adoption of a particular medium of interactional exchange, I have argued here, which can provide a feedback mechanism between the domains. Thus, through the situated use of conciliar rhetoric, 'The Young Yids' could accede to a collective trauma, become a group with both a public and a private face, while succeeding in remaining, as individuals, differentially motivated, attached and satisfied.[6]

NOTES

1 Income derives from the cod-fishery of the Grand Banks, as well as logging, mining and newly-found offshore oil deposits. However, the harsh climate, the distance from main markets, plus the smallness and scattered nature of the indigenous one and dependence on external investment, all eventuate in highly erratic (and seasonal) employment opportunities and an unemployment rate rising as high as 35 per cent (People's Commission, 1978).

2 Jokes dub Newfoundland 'Canada's Third World', claiming its backward population of 'Newfies' or 'Newfs' to be reliant upon mainland hand-outs and welfare initiatives.
3 As part of the 1949 Confederation agreement, this major ethnic division is still reflected in the religiously denominational schooling system: schools are run by the Roman Catholic School Board on the one side and by the Protestant Consolidated (Anglican, Presbyterian, Moravian, United and Salvation Army) or Pentecostal Boards on the other.
4 This quotation, later ones from *The Evening Telegram*, and the main interaction itself have had to be shortened due to limits on space.
5 In Austin's terms, conciliar rhetoric represents performative utterance (1975: 25; also cf. Bauman, 1978: 16).
6 For their comment and criticism on versions of this piece, my thanks go to Victor Zaslavsky, Robert Paine, Suzette Heald and Deborah Marks.

COMMENT

Dina Gertler

The organisation of a small restricted group was studied by Rapport, using what is known by psychologists as the 'systematic method' on verbal communication. He shows the development of a collective language of formal conciliar rhetoric which operates to legitimise the boundaries and status of the group. He concludes by showing how individual motivations permit a collective identity through ritualised forms of communication, which promote an identity which privileges the 'us' to the detriment of the 'me'. The group which is signified by the 'us' possesses both a public and a private face.

The research of Rapport is important from many points of view and especially because all studies of group formation can be looked at in this way. However, there is some doubt about whether Rapport's definition of ego-syntonism corresponds to the concept as developed by Devereux. That was based on the principle of complementarity and the mechanisms of subjective motivation. But verbal exchanges and conscious motivation cannot lead to the regressive mechanisms characteristic of group functioning at the level which is dominated by archaic fantasies. Fusion and primary sexuality cannot be understood by sticking to the overt discourse. According to A. Eiguer, beneath evident social exchanges one finds the distinctions of me/not me, body–space and the formation of object relationships among members. Winnicott thinks that the individual does not start out as a unitary being but that he constitutes himself by means of multiple identifications coming from his environment. Thus, the unity of self emerges only secondarily in social interaction, as a consequence of the intermediate space between inside and out, that is to say, of the 'transitional zone'. In the same way, for Devereux, what he refers to as ego-syntonism defines the articulation between social motives and subjective experience. In Rapport's paper, the psychic functions are ignored or reduced to an objective discourse.

How should one conceive of the dynamic between individual and the group functions? For Bion, this is done by means of a double repre-sentational and emotional function; instinct and fantasy are elaborated after the model of the new-born at the breast or upon a primal scene of partial objects. To my mind, the exclusion of sexuality in the group described by Rapport is a defence mechanism against archaic fantasies. It pertains to the exogamy of the 'family' group.

Through the reactionary formation, defensive isolation and the reinforcement of ethnic identity, the group of Young Yids define their relationship to Judaism in general and to the Jewish trauma in particular. From there, the family/group reconstructs its history over time: traumatic in the past, active in the present and with implications for the future. It is the collective trauma which provides the principal motive for the formation of the group.

The doubts raised by the revisionist newspaper on the reality of the Holocaust inflict a double trauma on these young Jewish Canadians. Its perverse statements constitute, on one side, a denial of the external historical reality and, on the other side, an attack on the internal reality and the work of mourning as it is lived in the families. It also constitutes an attack on the veracity of the memory, of a kind which threatens the sanity and mental stability of these more or less assimilated youths. The shock inflicted on these young people by this article reactivates the massive collective trauma in the unconscious part of their ethnic personality and reinforces, like a defensive reaction, their identity as a minority.

The psychoanalytic mind is slightly shocked by the idea proposed by the author that the gathering of individuals into a group allows them to keep at a distance or even exorcise the trauma, a view which ignores the inevit-ability of the work of mourning. For me, in this case, the coming together into a group constitutes a defensive action against a passive masochistic position. Naturally we stay there in the persecutory logic.

Time will make a difference between the lived trauma and that which has been transmitted; it is loaded with significance and its meanings will change. Subincision and circumcision are ethnic traumas which some cultures impose on their members and they carry symbolic value. But the Holocaust cannot be compared to such ethnic traumas because it is trauma external to the culture, absolute and non-symbolisable.

One might suppose that from now on, in the 'unconscious segment of the ethnic personality', Jewish and Gypsy, the mark of the trauma will persist, and that the external fact is transformed into an internal psychic structure, which is transmitted in the way that culture is transmitted through the super-ego of the parents. The exogenous trauma for the parents in this way becomes an endogenous trauma for their descendants. Clinical data confirm that the work of Sisyphus as it relates to mourning continues vertically through time. These processes have been described by Abraham and Torok (1976) in terms of internalised metaphors which are linked to failed introjections and liable to painful repetition.

RESPONSE

Nigel Rapport

Devereux quotes with approbation the 'Roman commonsense "psychologist" who pointed out that, "*Si bis faciunt idem, non est idem*" (if two people do the same thing, it is not the same thing)' (1978: 125). Devereux calls this a 'simple fact' but if he had written nothing else, his work would still be significant to me (if I have a regret, it is that Devereux found the quotation and used it as an epigraph first).

Devereux went further, however, and developed the notion of ego-syntonism, of different subjective meanings and motivations meeting in the same collective/objective act. The crucial dichotomy here, of course, is between public behaviour and its personal meaning, between collective action and its individual understanding (between what Georg Simmel would have identified as the commonality of form and the possible diversity of content). And this is, in turn, the motif that I seek to develop in my paper: how a number of actors can come together in a group, form a public collectivity and at precisely the same time stay apart and maintain their discrete and diverse individuality; indeed, how one enables the other: collectivity and individuality maintained through a constitutive tension of opposition.

I am not qualified to comment on Dr Gertler's description of the unconscious; I am prepared to accept that the ethnography I write can be made sense of within a psychoanalytic paradigm, but also that this in no way reduces the viability of what I would say regarding either individual cognition or symbolic interaction. As Devereux himself pointed out, explanations from within two (or more) paradigms, dealing with the 'same' explicandum – the mind, for example – can be compatible, 'complementary' and, in their own terms, both valid. Indeed, such a 'double discourse', the locating of a phenomenon within two (or more) explanatory perspectives, is 'mandatory', 'inevitable', to 'prove that the phenomenon is real'; while neither paradigm or perspective is reducible to, or circumscribable by – even enunciable by – the other (1978: 1). In other words, the same objective phenomenon (public exchange between The Newfoundland Young Yids about the Holocaust) provides an ego-syntonic outlet for the gratification of at least two paradigmatic motivations. Which, of course, brings me back to the point of my paper: *'Dina Schwartz': 'Basil LaRusic':: Dina Gertler: Nigel Rapport.*

More precisely, if Dr Gertler believes that in groups, individuals 'regress' so that identities fuse, boundaries between selves and between bodies collapse, and 'archaic fantasies' and 'part objects' dominate, then, equally, I believe that in groups individuals have no better environment through which to hide and yet maintain their self-identities. Individuals may be never more completely themselves than in groups: groups represent the perfect public guise for individuality. And the key to this, I would agree, is not to take the group's shared, 'manifest discourse' at face value: individuals may partake superficially but ultimately subvert this, if not cognitively absenting themselves altogether.

Again, if Dr Gertler believes that there is a 'collective Jewish trauma' which provides the impetus towards the formation of The Y.Y./The Soviet Jewry Action Council (when the denial of the Holocaust attacks an inevitable, ongoing 'family mourning process' and thus threatens these youths' 'sanity and mental stability'), a trauma, indeed, whose 'persecutive logic', 'externality' and 'absoluteness' no 'symbolic defensive action' can alleviate, then, equally, I believe that there is no reality which is 'non-symbolisable'. That is, the trauma of the Holocaust is a symbol, sufficiently public, dominant, even clichéd for these youths to use it as a simple excuse, as a manifestly obvious reason for their coming together; they draw on its publicity, its conventionality, so that, for a moment, in the situation of being 'Newfoundland Young Yids', they can act as Jews, as serious and responsible adults, as familiar and familial, as historically and corporately linked to an Old World religious tradition. The Holocaust, in short, is a sacred symbol which provides these individuals with the ego-syntonic opportunity at once to belong, to embrace (and reverse) a stigmatised, collective identity, and at the same time to construct personal experiences which are varied, idiosyncratic and momentary; as with any other instance of symbolic usage, they try the cliché on for size.

I agree that the individual is a being of 'multiple' and not 'unitary identification', even while the individual might still have occasion to think of himself as 'a unity'. But it is not a question, for me, of one being 'primary' and one 'emerging secondarily'; nor of individual self-identification as something which simply 'comes from his environment' and 'articulates' with the latter's changes. The individual remains multiple: he creates a number of identities for himself and situates these in a number of social worlds. Indeed, these worlds are so full and complex that when

94 Complementarity

cognitively situated in any one of them, all eventualities, past and present, can be understood in those terms: the individual feels he has always been this one thinking person and always will be. But, most significantly, the ongoing initiative of understanding is his, the agency and creativity of interpretation remain his. Thus, the context of individual action must also be understood as something internal to individual consciousness: a matter of self-placement, limited only by his imagination, as George Kelly (1969) phrased it; here is a personal decision concerning the characteristics and the situationality of public space. Moreover, the individual must empathise hard (and guess lucky) if he wishes his interpretation and that of others to overlap. For far more likely will be the moments of ego-syntonism: meetings of public form rather than personal content.

I am very grateful to Dina Gertler for her critical remarks, as well as to Suzette Heald, Deborah Marks and Henrietta Moore for their translation and elucidation.

BIBLIOGRAPHY

Abraham, N. and Torok, M. (1976) *Le Verbier de l'homme aux loups*. Paris: Editions Aubier.
Austin, J. L. (1975) *How to Do Things with Words*. Oxford: Clarendon Press.
Bailey, F. G. (1965) 'Decisions by consensus in councils and committees; with special reference to village and local government in India', in ASA Monographs no.2, *Political Systems and the Distribution of Power*. London: Tavistock.
Bauman, R. (1978) *Verbal Art as Performance*. Rowley: Newbury House.
Bernstein, B. (1964) 'Aspects of language and learning in the genesis of social process', in D. Hymes (ed.) *Language in Culture and Society*. New York: Harper & Row.
—— (1972) 'A sociolinguistic approach to socialisation; with some reference to educability', in J. Gumperz and D. Hymes (eds) *Directions in Sociolinguistics*. New York: Holt, Rinehart & Winston.
Devereux, G. (1978) *Ethnopsychoanalysis*. Berkeley: University of California Press.
Evening Telegram, The (1985) 23 February and 2 March. 400 Topsail Rd, St John's.
Gal, S. (1989) 'Language and political economy', *Annual Review of Anthropology* 18: 345–67.
Gilad, L. (1989) *The Northern Route*. St John's: ISER Press, Memorial University.
Hook, R. H. (ed.) (1979) *Fantasy and Symbol: Studies in Anthropological Interpretation*. London: Academic Press.
Kahn, A. (1987) *Listen While I Tell You: A Story of the Jews of Newfoundland*. St John's: ISER Press, Memorial University.
Kelly, G. (1969) *Clinical Psychology and Personality: The Selected Papers of George Kelly*, ed. B. Maher. New York: Wiley.
Kuper, A. (1971) 'Council structure and decision-making', in A. Richards and A. Kuper (eds) *Councils in Action*. Cambridge: Cambridge University Press.
Paine, R. (1976) 'Two modes of exchange and mediation', in B. Kapferer (ed.) *Transaction and Meaning*. Philadelphia: ISHI.

People's Commission on Unemployment (1978) *'Now that We've Burned our Boats . . .'*. St John's: Newfoundland and Labrador Federation of Labour.

Rapport, N. J. (1986) 'Cedar High Farm: ambiguous symbolic boundary. An essay in anthropological intuition', in A. P. Cohen (ed.) *Symbolising Boundaries: Identity and Diversity in British Cultures*. Manchester: Manchester University Press.

—— (1987) *Talking Violence: An Anthropological Interpretation of Conversation in the City*. St John's: ISER Press.

—— (1988) 'A policeman's construction of "the truth": Sergeant Hibbs and the lie-detector machine', *Anthropology Today* 4: 7–11.

—— (1990) 'Ritual conversation in a Canadian suburb: anthropology and the problem of generalisation', *Human Relations* 43: 849–64.

Richards, A. (1971) 'The nature of the problem', in A. Richards and A. Kuper (eds) *Councils in Action*. Cambridge: Cambridge University Press.

Part II
The analysis of dreams

6 Dream imagery becomes social experience

The cultural elucidation of dream interpretation[1]

Iain Edgar

Dreaming is a universal aspect of being human. It appears to be the most private and hidden activity which is usually perceived as being both unpredictable and often incomprehensible. Yet most human societies have sought to understand dream imagery and many have accorded such imagery and its interpretations high, even prophetic, significance. The paradoxical and ambivalent position of the dream is well illustrated in western industrialised societies where, on the one hand, 'interpreting dreams' is seen as a highly specialised task reserved for psychoanalysts and needing a long and challenging training. On the other hand, dreaming is denigrated as being wholly illusory, as being just a 'dream' and of no consequence.

Tedlock (1987a) has traced the origin of western disregard of the value of dreaming back to Aristotelian scholasticism. The development of Cartesian dualism in the seventeenth century set the seal on the relegation of dream imagery to the realm of the unreal. The 'oppositional dichotomy' (Tedlock, 1987a: 2) thus erected between subjective and objective reality, reality and unreality, meant the exclusion of dreaming from serious consideration in the west until the twentieth century. Freud's development of psychoanalysis, his use of dream imagery and his conceptualisation of the unconscious clearly started a new era in terms of the evaluation of the dream. Such a historical and negative evaluation of the dream is not however universal. In the Indian Hindu tradition dreaming is placed above waking reality in the hierarchy of realities (Tedlock, 1987a: 3). In the Islamic Sufi tradition a form of reality is identified which is midway between sensibility and spirituality. This is identified by Corbin (1966) as the 'imaginal world' which is an autonomous world of imagery and forms accessible through both dreaming and techniques of active imagination (Price-Williams, 1987). Moreover, outside the great world religious traditions there is abundant evidence from anthropologists to show that many non-industrialised societies value and use dream imagery as part of their participatory experience of reality (Tylor, 1871; Firth, 1934; Devereux, 1951; Hallowell, 1966; Tedlock, 1987a; Herdt, 1987; Mannheim, 1987).

Indeed, the current situation regarding the evaluation of the dream in westernised societies is even more perplexing when we try to differentiate between 'vision' and 'dream'. Whereas a 'dream' can be discounted as 'just a dream', 'vision', whether that of the leader or manager, is highly regarded as a core ability. Sometimes there is even a conflation of these two terms as when Martin Luther King started his famous speech by saying 'I have a dream . . .'. Such examples well illustrate our social ambivalence about 'the pictures in our mind', or mental imagery.

While there is evidently laxity in the referential meaning of the word 'dream', in this paper I am generally using the term to describe the particular mental imagery experienced in sleep. My particular interest is in illustrating a process of transformation that is at the heart of dream interpretation and which sheds light upon the nature of our understanding of both self and world. The process of transformation I am referring to is that between the perceived internal image – the dream image – of the dreamer and its translation into a social and personal meaning for the individual dreamer.

Dream interpretation then consists of several stages. There is the recollection of the dream by the dreamer and then the subsequent filtering of the original imagery into what Kracke (1987) describes as 'language-centred thought processes'. This filtration of imagery into thought is an act of translation which begins the construction of meaning by the relating of the visual imagery to the cognitive categories of the culture of the dreamer. Such cognitive categories carry implicit ways of ordering and sequencing time and space, person and action that inevitably begin to define the possible readings of the text or narration. Brown (1987: 155) presents this translation through the Freudian distinction between primary and second-ary process thinking, arguing that dream imagery is immediately translated from primary process thinking into secondary process thinking upon recollection. The dream audience can receive only the verbal text of the dream even if that text is embellished by drawings and paintings of the dream imagery. Often the dream narration is already the beginning of an interpretative process in so far as the dreamer will be associating with the sensory imagery. The dream has then become a text available to an audience, and as such is open to a hermeneutic analysis (Ricoeur, 1970), though Kracke (1987) criticises such an approach in its entirety as it negates the continued involvement of the dreamer with the dream imagery during the interpretive process.

The dream narration itself is a social act which both expresses and creates social affinity and meaning. There is still a gap between thought and speech. Herdt (1987) uses the idea of discourse frames to express this perception. In the Sambian society of New Guinea, Herdt found three different discourses within which dream sharing took place. There was public talk, secret talk and private talk. Each of these discourses was structured in differing ways in relation to 'cultural rules, premises, expectations – frames that organise behaviour'. Public discourse was the most common discourse in which anyone in the social group could be present. Secret discourse referred to the communication of ritual secrets and was sexually segregated. Private discourse concerned personal secrets typically about sexuality. The question of the importance of knowing which parts of dreams are not being shared is clearly demonstrated in this example. An entertaining incident from one of my studied dreamwork groups was when the group split into three small groups of three or four members to discuss recent dreams. One group was composed of three women and each coincidentally shared a recent dream involving faeces and with much laughter admitted in the feedback to the larger group that had they not been in the small, same-gender group they would not have shared that dream content. Examples of group members not disclosing sexual contents of dream images, particularly when they referred to other group members, were commonplace and emerged in the subsequent individual interviews. The not-narrated can then be as significant as the narrated! Such examples show how important knowledge of group and social processes is to the interpretation of disclosed dreams.

The history of anthropological interest in dreaming has until recently been focused on the narration of the dream and has tended to avoid the cultural context of the narration. From the 1920s to the 1960s anthropologists were concerned with a Freudian-based analysis of cross-cultural dream material and the search for transcultural psychological patterning to dreams. Seligman's (1924) search for common latent meaning to dream material and especially the content analysis school of dream analysis (Hall, 1951; Eggan, 1952; Hall and Van de Castle, 1966) are prime examples of such approaches. Sociologists such as Bastide (1966) have viewed dreams as both expressing and trying to resolve the conflicts of each society. In particular he tried to show how the oppressive experience of marginalised groups was vividly presented and reconstructed in their dreams. By the 1970s dreamwork was beginning to be considered within the cultural system of which it was a part. Crapanzano (1975) analysed the metaphorical usage of saints and jinns in the dreamworld of the Moroccan Hamadsha. He showed that personal use of particular dream symbols and their performative function in terms of conflict recognition and possible solution were firmly embedded within the 'implicit folk psychology' or 'psychological idiom' of the culture. More recently, anthropologists have continued to develop the concept of the dream report. Tedlock (1987a: 25) suggested that the manifest dream content 'should be expanded to include more than the dream report. Ideally it should include dream theory or theories and ways of sharing, including the relevant discourse frames, and the cultural code for dream interpretation.'

Tedlock describes this perspective as a communicative theory of dreaming. This theory would consider the dream narration as a communicative event involving the act and creation of narration, the psychodynamics of narration and the emic interpretative framework. Such a theory would consider dream analysis as more than a hermeneutically based textual analysis; rather as a social and cultural process or activity that would have both expressive and instrumental outcomes. When this takes place then, as Herdt (1987) writes, we may take seriously the proposition 'that culture may actually change experience inside of dreams, or that the productions of dreaming do actually become absorbed and transfomed into culture'.

Such a communicative theory of dreaming alerts us to the importance of the psychodynamics of the social setting and the interpretative framework of the participants. The social anthropologist is then concerned with the analysis of this interpretative framework which necessarily structures the narration and interpretation. Two examples from Tedlock's edited volume (Tedlock, 1987a) and one example from my research will illustrate this important point.

Basso (1987) relates her analysis of the dream theory of the Kalapalo Indians of Central Brazil to the differences between Freudian and Jungian perspectives on dreaming. Freud related dream imagery to the past whereas Jung saw such imagery as possible symbolic sketches of the dreamer's future. Jung (1948: 255) called this a prospective function of dreams, not to be confused with a prophetic function. Basso saw as progressive those emic theories of dreaming that understood that dream imagery is future orientated in so far as the dreamer uses dream imagery and its symbolisation of current concerns to speculate upon and orientate to future goals of the self. In this way Tedlock (1987b) compared the different ways of dream sharing and dream interpretation between two Mexican and Guatemalan groups, the Zuni and the Quiche, to show how such differences are rooted in contrasting metaphysical and psychological systems. How the living and the deceased are differentially conceptualised is crucial in her analysis.

The emic dream theory of the group may not however be singular and consensual. Dream theory can be multi-variant and contradictory, as with the psychodynamic tradition in westernised societies. In the dreamwork groups that I ran and which I will introduce shortly, the key interpretative difference was in relation to the acceptability of a well-known part of the Freudian paradigm. There was a split in the group between members who tended to want to interpret dream imagery as covert sexual symbols and those who felt that they were well able to dream explicitly of sexual issues when necessary and resented such sexual interpretations of their imagery. An example of this was a female group member having a dream of 'another woman having a gynaecological operation, lying in a tank of water. One of the doctors was carrying a huge hypodermic syringe and injected it into the woman's skull.' The issue of another female group member interpreting this image as a sexual one was still unresolved weeks later when the original dreamer angrily disclosed to the group that there had been a subsequent and sexually explicit progression in the dream that she had not previously disclosed. The dreamer disclosed this additional information to show to the group that she was able to dream explicitly about sexual matters and to invalidate the suggestion that the hypodermic was a covert sexual symbol. This example also illustrated contemporaneously the importance of non-narration or, in this case, delayed narration of sensitive dream data.

So far we have demonstrated a process of translation in our understanding of dream interpretation that involves the following sequence: emic dream theory–dream–dream narration–psychodynamics of dream audience–interpretative process–relating of interpretation to future of self and group. This final stage of relating interpretation to the future of the dreamer or group will be shown in my own research data and is illustrated by Basso's progressive theory of dreaming. However, this account obscures two further aspects or even stages of this translation process. These are the social construction of the dream data themselves and their interpretation via the group reflection on the metaphorical nature of language itself.

DREAMWORK GROUPS

In the next section I aim to show how the rather obvious point that people dream within the symbolic idiom of their particular culture was reflected in certain dreams from the groups I studied. I also hope to show that part of the interpretative process was derived from a metaphorical analysis of the meaning of ordinary language use. Thus I will complete the process of showing how dream imagery can be perceived as an intense and affective form of metaphorical thought that is culturally derived from the symbolic forms of the particular society. Moreover, this dream imagery can be and has been found to be meaningful within the prevailing systems of meaning in language. We will then see a complete circle of transformation in which dream imagery is both socially constructed and socially interpreted by means of cultural symbolism.

The genesis of this dreamwork group and the associated research lies in my own long-standing interest in and occasional 'use'of my own personal dream imagery. For over twenty years I have often been struck by the ability of dream imagery to reformulate imaginatively situations that were preoccupying my waking thoughts. These reformulations, although often bizarre, sometimes seemed to have an anticipatory aspect to them, rather as Basso has suggested. I found that occasionally, by dwelling on a seemingly powerful dream image and by turning it around in my mind and considering how it might relate to developing situations in my life, I was able to arrive at a conclusion. Such a conclusion often took the form of a decision about the direction of my life with respect to, for instance, career development or relationship issues. I then considered that the process I was conducting was a more explicit formulation of the folk wisdom advice to 'sleep on it' if one had a difficult problem to mull over. So for several years I kept a dream diary and consciously tried to remember my dreams. At this time I immersed myself in the work of Jung and realised that he had similarly advocated such a significant relationship to one's dream imagery. By significant he meant that it was insufficient to relate to dream imagery solely as a kind of internalised source of artwork, but that, through a dialogue with one's dream imagery, important insights might emerge that could lead to personal change and development.

What was, off and on, a personal interest developed in two ways. Firstly, I encountered the dreamwork movement in the mid-1980s through participation as a member in a personal development group that included a consideration of dreams. This particular group combined bodywork exercises, meditation and discussion of members' dream imagery. The dreamwork movement itself began in the 1970s in the USA as an offshoot of the human potential or personal growth movement. At this time the publication of works by authors such as Garfield (1974) and Ullman and Zimmerman (1979) both popularised and guided groups and individuals into ways of working with their dreams. The dreamwork movement values dream imagery as being of potential benefit to the dreamer and the 'meaning' of such imagery as being accessible and understandable to the interested person (Hillman, 1989). Dreamwork groups are relatively commonplace in the USA but are less frequent in the UK. Through the group that I participated in I became interested in the linking of group process to the understanding of dream material. Secondly, while researching a therapeutic community (Edgar, 1986), I experienced a significant sequence of dreams just before, during and after the fieldwork stage. I found that contemplating these images and wondering how they might relate to the fieldwork experience was a powerful source of insight, assisted in my orientation to the varying stages of the fieldwork process and imaginatively pre-figured core themes of my research (Edgar, 1989).

The publication of Tedlock's edited volume on contemporary anthropological approaches to dreamwork both re-established the cultural analysis of dreamwork as part of the anthropological enterprise and showed me that there was a dearth of data about the cultural aspects of dreamwork in advanced industrial societies. Then, at the same time, it became evident from my contacts that there were a number of people who had an interest in dreaming and in interpreting dream imagery in a group context. The idea of establishing a dreamwork group thus had a dual aim: both to facilitate dream interpretation in a group context for therapeutic purposes and, at the same time, to study this process.

The experience of dreamwork groups that I will now draw on consists of co-leading three ten-week groups of approximately two to two-and-a-half hours' duration. These happened between September 1989 and June 1990. Recruitment to the group was by local advertising, word of mouth and through the membership networks of the local independent groupwork training agency where the sessions were held. The recruitment literature suggested only that potential group members should be interested in sharing their dreams. We did not interview or select members prior to the start of the first session of each of the three groups. The room we used was distinctive in that there were no chairs but only a number of large cushions. Group size was between six and twelve.

The first group had six members of whom four continued till the end of the third group. The second group contained twelve people which was really too big and the third group contained nine members. On average, one person started each of the three groups but left after one or two sessions. Members were of all ages but were mainly female, white and professional. Some were married but most were separated or divorced and with children of varying ages. Several members knew each other previously either through groupwork or circle dancing weekends. Many of the members had interests in what very loosely could be described as New Age pursuits such as yoga, meditation, astrology, circle dancing[2] and aromatherapy. However, while most or all members had been to therapy or personal growth groups before, none had been to dreamwork groups. Apart from two members who attended Quaker meetings and one who was a Methodist, mainstream religious commitments were not evident.

Almost all the members who stayed through a group term of ten weeks disclosed either to the group or in the follow-up interviews that they were going through a period of their life which involved, in their eyes, great change or considerable crisis. These crises were typical of the crises of our times, that is ageing, separation, divorce and work/career stress. Whether the magnitude of these perceived changes differed from the scale of life change normally experienced it is not possible to say. However, it became clear that the years following, for instance, a marriage break up could still contain a major sequence of 'coming to terms' with the loss and change experienced. Indeed, the conscious processing of these change experiences in relation to the recalled dream imagery provided the bulk of the subject matter of the group discussions.

There were two co-leaders, myself and a female colleague who was a freelance groupworker and counsellor. As group leaders or facilitators we prioritised the telling of and the working with members' dreams and tended to disclose our own dreams only once on average during a ten-week session. These occasions were when either no member had a dream or, in my case, it was the final week of a group term. There was a level of groupwork expertise and some members were well able to facilitate gestalt and psychodramatic exercises for example. However, several members were not so experienced and exhibited reluctance and shyness in relationship to the disclosure of both the detail and form of personal concerns.

While one might expect a high level of cohesion given a relatively sophisticated group membership, this did not preclude significant differences and conflicts emerging at different times. Such differences were, for example, around the centrality of dreamwork in the sessions and related to some members' wish to spend more time on non-dream-related personal issues. Another focus of occasional discontent was around the nature of interpretative comment by members and, in particular, as we have already seen, whether a sexual interpretation of dream imagery was to be prioritised by the group. In the event, a core of eight group members continued after the finish of the three-term programme and have constituted a self-directed dreamwork group for the last two years.

The group programme usually consisted of a structured round at the beginning in which members talked about their personal situation and feelings, gave a short description of any dream they had and said if they wanted to work on it. Then the group would choose two or three dreams to consider during the rest of the evening. The most common method of working with a dream was by suggestion, discussion, association and comparison. The group attempted to help the dreamer relate their dream imagery to their current daytime, conscious life. We regularly supplemented discussion with action techniques such as the use of gestalt exercises, particularly on emotional identification with different parts of the dream, psychodrama, artwork, meditation and visualisation. The visualisation exercises proved particularly productive and were always based on a powerful image from a member's dreams. Images used in visualisation ranged from 'being a bulb' to 'going on a journey as a bird' to visualising a 'door in the mind' and then going through it. Every session was audiotaped for research purposes and members had access to the tapes.

I will now present three examples of dreamwork, mainly from the first group. Anonymity will be preserved through minor changes to place and person. I will try to distinguish three interacting levels within the analysis, that of the personal, the group and the cultural. The first dream image I will discuss is that of a woman who had sherry glasses in her hair as hair rollers! This was part of a longer dream involving a walk in the country with a male friend and seeing a kind of Victorian theatre performance in a barn. During the session the woman did a gestalt identification with 'being the sherry glass' and talking to the group from that imaginative position. On a personal level, feelings of fragility, age, being valued and long used sprang up through this exercise. These were immediately related by her to her current emotional situation of coping with recent divorce and separation. Issues of power and the use that is made of someone were facilitated through later discussion, as were current feelings about herself. Personal meaning of the hair symbol was sought through spontaneous association and insight into metaphorical language use such as the sexualised meaning of 'letting your hair down'. The dreamer later related her hair image to the Samson myth of the vitality and strength of hair.

On a group level there was, firstly, a humorous preoccupation with the gendered sexual symbolism of the sherry glass and its being filled with golden liquid contents and, secondly, an awareness by female members of their 'being used' by other people, particularly men. On a social level we can see perhaps a rather class- and gender-based appropriation of the sherry glass symbol both within the dream narration and the subsequent interpretive process. The female is defined as a passive and decorative container who exists for the pleasure and gratification of others, usually men, who will fill and enrich her emptiness. The use of the Samson and Delilah myth can fix female sexual power within an imaginative order that affirms male virility and feminine deceit.

The dialogue between personal image and potential social meaning as evidenced in the metaphors of ordinary language, such as in 'letting your hair down', became a feature of group members 'making sense' of their dream imagery, as will be further shown in the next example.

The next dream reflects another woman's concern with her current job situation and an impending interview. The dream in summary concerned this woman going for interview in a bookshop. She was carrying a large loaf of bread in her arms. There was icing on top of the bread which suddenly started to drip off. Her ex-partner and his girlfriend were also there. The unpacking of meanings from this dream imagery was long and complex and involved the member reflecting on her present job situation and feelings about current and past key relationships. Overall, the dream reflected her anxiety and fear of assessment linked to a present fragility of self-image in the domestic sphere. By doing a gestalt identification with the icing on the bread she got in contact with very basic feelings and perceptions about her mother and her mother's expectations of her. Throughout the discussion and exercise a powerful theme for the group was the spontaneous discovery of the various metaphors of bread embedded in ordinary language use such as 'using your loaf', being 'kneaded', being 'proved', 'being good enough to eat', a 'bun in the oven' and 'loafing about'. These became both humorous asides and also powerful metaphorical summaries, via the puns on, for example, 'being needed' and 'being proved', of the dreamer's self-state and current self-image. She, during this session, developed an identification with the bread symbol which became a multi-vocal symbol of the self capable of many different amplifications of meaning.

Such meanings are derived from this dialogue between self and group, and elicited by reflecting on how we derive our dream imagery from our culture, and then in turn understanding our dream imagery by considering the use of metaphor in everyday language.

While the group in this session was focused on assisting the dreamer narrator and playing with these 'bread' metaphors, the issues arising from the discussion again are reflective of structural, in this case patriarchal, aspects of culture. The dreamer identified the linking of the bread and the icing and the interview with her concern about maintaining her physical attractiveness and avoiding her male partner's rejection if she became overweight. The group on this occasion focused on affirming the innate attractiveness of the dreamer, without reference to male expectation, and the ability of the dreamer to define herself – to become 'her own loaf'!

The third example is a 'button' dream. In part of this dream another female member reported a dream of a beautiful art deco button in a shop and herself as having a button hanging loose from her coat. Discussion of this dream led on to the woman revealing major life preoccupations. The art deco button came to represent the dreamer's conflict between clothing and dress accessories as being for display or for utility. Latent feelings of having always to meet her own needs last and feelings of low self-esteem were expressed. She identified the loose button as representing a much greater impending personal loss in her life, that of her partner. As in the other two dreams, the button symbol's potency was explored through the spontaneous consideration of the idiomatic usage of the 'button' and 'thread' symbols, as in such phrases as 'bright as a button', 'buttoned up', 'unbuttoned' and 'hanging by a thread'. At a social level the revealed interpersonal and sexual symbolism of buttons in this culture became a vehicle for developing personal understanding. Such a discussion of both learnt and experienced symbolism again gave the group the opportunity to reflect critically on questions of gender roles, socialisation and opportunities for empowerment by women.

Through the brief examples from these three dream narrations and discussions we can see how the dreamer and the group use significantly gendered
and sexual symbols both unconsciously in dream material and consciously in
group dialogue. The examples show that dream data consist of sets and
sequences of images that are derived from everyday life and can reflect current
concerns of the dreamer. While it is possible to understand dream imagery as
a particular form of mentation without meaning, such as a cognitive-
psychological approach asserts (Foulkes, 1985), there is a strong collective
human tradition which seeks to find meaning in dream imagery. Kracke (1987:
38) defines Freud's notion of the dream as primary process thought in terms of
'a highly condensed, visual or sensory, metaphorical form of thinking'. He
suggests that the dream, like the myth for Lévi-Strauss, is a kind of *bricolage*
in that it gathers 'from among the day residues ready to hand, and uses them to
express metaphorically an emotional conflict, and to work out (or work
toward) some resolution of it' (Kracke, 1987: 38). Such a view of the value and
role of dreaming is congruent with a 'revised psychoanalytic perspective'
(Gluckman and Warner, 1987) in which the traditional Freudian-based distinction between primary and secondary process thought and the distinction
between the manifest and latent meanings of the dream have been re-
evaluated. Dreaming in this neo-Freudian perspective is seen rather as a
manifest problem solving and the integrative process that takes place as
metaphorical thought.

The dream can then be seen as a form of metaphorical thought. The
ultimate question as to whether 'dreams' have meaning is currently un-
answerable, though laboratory research into the significance of REM sleep
appears to show that subjects need to make up any 'lost' REM sleep
(Tedlock, 1987a: 12). What is clear is that many peoples, including the
sample I studied in the dreamwork group, create and have created an
understanding of their dreams which they could relate to their current
personal life.

METAPHOR AND THE SOCIAL RELEVANCE OF
DREAMWORK

The dream is however not the only form of metaphorical thought. Lakoff
and Johnson (1980) have analysed the metaphorical basis of our rationality
and language. They have shown how our conceptual system is fundamentally metaphorical in nature and that metaphor implicitly structures our
consciousness and action. Metaphor works by 'understanding and
experiencing one kind of thing in terms of another' (Lakoff and Johnson,
1980: 5). Moreover, the metaphors that structure our consciousness are
based on our everyday experience and are not arbitrary. For instance, there

is a relationship between our experience of spatial living, the 'spatial/ orientational metaphors' such as 'up/down' and human states of wellbeing and sickness. States of happiness tend to be expressed as 'being up' in some form and likewise being dejected or sad is commonly metaphorically described as being 'down' in some way, as in the phrase 'I'm feeling down'. There is then a continuing dialogue and relationship between our physical and cultural experience and our understanding of the world through a metaphorically structured language-centred consciousness. We can then postulate that metaphorical thought is the basis of both dream imagery and conscious awareness. No wonder then that the two are linked! As Bourdieu says, 'the mind is a metaphor of the world of objects which is itself but an endless circle of mutually reflecting metaphors' (1977: 91). Further, we have seen how the insights generated by the group's reflection on the dream data are created and validated through the relating of these data to the metaphorical meanings contained in ordinary language usage.

Moreover, these socially constructed systems of meaning are continually being re-evaluated, as can be seen in the following example drawn from a family therapist recently writing about using dreamwork in such therapy. Buchholz (1990) analysed examples of using dream material in family therapy situations. He encountered a deep level of mutual understanding of dreams within these families. In one example both the 18-year-old boy, Billy, and his father had had the same dream in which Billy was pursued out of a cellar by a witch figure. Discussion of this dream image opened up key dynamics within the family linking Billy's drug addiction to his relationship to and between his parents. The 'witch' image was chronologically and dynamically linked to an early description of Billy's mother by her mother-in-law as being a 'witch', and overall the dream was understood in the session as expressing Billy's wish to escape a seductive mother. This 'witch' image appears to have been a key for both the male and female members of this family to disclose deep fears and hitherto unrevealed fantasy material about each other. Interestingly, the negative meaning ascribed to the 'witch' image in the discussion about the dream is presented in the article as being unproblematic. Yet, such a negative stereotyping or interpretation of the 'witch' image can be critiqued from a feminist perspective as being a deeply sexist interpretation. Such a conflictual diversity of interpretation well illustrates the micro-cultural and political aspects of contemporary dreamwork. Likewise the feminist interpretations evident in the examples from my dream data similarly illustrate the point.

Finally, this analysis brings up the question of the potential use of this kind of mental imagery as a way of understanding social life. In this paper I have shown examples of how people have come to understand, and interpret within a group context, their dream imagery. These examples illustrate the cultural specificity of dream imagery and dream interpretation, and offer insight into the social construction of both the unconscious and the interpretative process itself. Furthermore, the examples illustrate the problem-solving capacity of dream imagery and dreamwork, as well as exemplifying the metaphorical nature of cognition and language.

Finally, a further development this decade has seen is the beginning of the use of both the researcher's and the informants' dreams for ethnographic research purposes. In particular, such dreams can throw light on the subjective orientation and cultural position of the anthropologist, as well as on the intersubjective encounter between anthropologist and informant. As Hastrup (1992: 119) has written, 'all ethnographers are positioned subjects and grasp certain phenomena better than others', so a reflexive anthropology may well come to consider dream imagery a valuable source of insight as well as a way to examine critically the progress of the fieldwork enterprise. Levine (1981) analysed the dreams of three of her informants for transference material concerning her relationship with these informants. She was able to gain an increased awareness of issues such as power, asymmetry between herself and informants, about poverty and dependence and about the degree of gender support she was offering to one of her informants during their marital difficulties. I have tried (Edgar, 1989) to relate my dreams experienced during fieldwork to both the stages of fieldwork research and the eventual analytic themes that developed in my master's thesis (1986). Hillman (1989: 137) has also recently suggested that dreams can provide the ethnographer with important insights into emotional and conflictual aspects of their fieldwork situation. Whether the anthropological study of the 'other' will necessarily one day embrace the researcher's own unconscious has yet to be seen, though Caplan (1988: 17) has suggested, in her discussion of 'engendering knowledge' that:

> the time has come for us all, male and female, to recognise that the sense of self which has sustained the practice of ethnography for so long is irrelevant and that as the French poet Rimbaud put it '*Je est un autre*'.

NOTES

1 A first draft of this chapter was given at the 1992 European Association of Social Anthropology Conference in Prague in a workshop titled 'Social Experience and Anthropological Knowledge'. I am very grateful to the workshop organisers Kirsten Hastrup and Peter Hervik for their initial invitation and their subsequent supportive comments.
2 Circle dancing is a form of folk dancing for small groups derived from European folk dance traditions and involving movement in either circle or line formations.

BIBLIOGRAPHY

Basso, E. B. (1987) 'The implications of a progressive theory of dreaming', in B. Tedlock (ed.) *Dreaming: Anthropological and Psychological Interpretations.* Cambridge: Cambridge University Press.

Bastide, R. (1966) 'Sociology of the dream', in V. Grunebaum and R. Caillois (eds) *The Dream and Human Societies.* Berkeley: University of California Press.

Bourdieu, P. (1977) *Outline of a Theory of Practice.* Cambridge: Cambridge University Press.

Brown, M. F. (1987) 'Ropes of sand: order and imagery in Aquaruna dreams', in B. Tedlock (ed.) *Dreaming: Anthropological and Psychological Interpretations.* Cambridge: Cambridge University Press.

Buchholz, M. B. (1990) 'Using dreams in family therapy', *Journal of Family Therapy* 12: 4.

Caplan, P. (1988) 'Engendering knowledge: the politics of ethnography (Part 2)', *Anthropology Today* 4(6):14–17.

Corbin, H. (1966) 'The visionary dream in Islamic spirituality', in G. Von Grunebaum and R. Callois (eds) *The Dream in Human Societies.* Berkeley: University of California Press.

Crapanzano, V. (1975) 'Saints, Jnun, and dreams: an essay in Moroccan ethnopsychiatry', *Psychiatry* 38: 145–59.

Devereux, G. (1951) *Reality and Dream: The Psychotherapy of a Plains Indian.* New York: International Universities Press.

Edgar, I. R. (1986) 'An anthropological analysis of Peper Harow therapeutic community with particular reference to the use of myth, ritual and symbol', unpublished M.Phil. thesis, University of Durham.

—— (1989) 'Dreaming as ethnography', unpublished paper given at the Association of Social Anthropologists Annual Conference in York, England.

Eggan, D. (1952) 'The manifest content of dreams: a challenge to social sciences', *American Anthropologist* 54: 469–85.

Firth, R. (1934) 'The meaning of dreams in Tikopia', in E. E. Evans-Pritchard (ed.) *Essays Presented to C. G. Seligman.* London: Kegan Paul.

Foulkes, D. (1985) *Dreaming: A Cognitive-Psychological Analysis.* London: Lawrence Erlbaum.

Garfield, P. (1974) *Creative Dreaming.* New York: Ballantine.

Gluckman, M. L and Warner, S. L. (1987) *Dreams in New Perspective.* New York: Human Sciences Press.

Hall, C. (1951) 'What people dream about', *Scientific American* 184: 60–3.

Hall, C. and Van De Castle, R. (1966) *The Content Analysis of Dreams.* New York: New American Library.

Hallowell, A. (1966) 'The role of the dream in Ojibwa culture', in G. Von Grunebaum and R. Callois (eds) *The Dream and Human Societies.* Berkeley: University of California Press.

Hastrup, K. (1992) 'Writing ethnography: state of the art', in J. Okely and H. Callaway (eds) *Anthropology and Autobiography.* London: Routledge.

Herdt, G. (1987) 'Selfhood and discourse in Sambia dream sharing', in B. Tedlock (ed.) *Dreaming: Anthropological and Psychological Interpretations.* Cambridge: Cambridge University Press.

Hillman, D. L. (1989) 'Dreamwork and fieldwork: linking cultural anthropology and the current dreamwork movement', in M. Ullman and C. Limmer (eds) *The Variety of Dream Experience*. Wellingborough: Aquarian Press.

Jung, C. G. (1948) 'General aspects of dream psychology', *Collected Works*, Vol. 8. London: Routledge.

Kracke, W. (1987) 'Myths in dreams, thought in images: an Amazonian contribution to the psychoanalytic theory of primary process', in B. Tedlock (ed.) *Dreaming: Anthropological and Psychological Interpretations*. Cambridge: Cambridge University Press.

Lakoff, G. and Johnson, M. (1980) *Metaphors We Live By*. Chicago: University of Chicago Press.

Levine, S. (1981) 'Dreams of the informant about the researcher: some difficulties inherent in the research relationship', *Ethos* 9: 276–93.

Mannheim, B. (1987) 'A semiotic of Andean dreams', in B. Tedlock (ed.) *Dreaming: Anthropological and Psychological Interpretations*. Cambridge: Cambridge University Press.

Price-Williams, D. (1987) 'The waking dream in ethnographic perspective', in B. Tedlock (ed.) *Dreaming: Anthropological and Psychological Interpretations*. Cambridge: Cambridge University Press.

Ricoeur, P. (1970) *Freud and Philosophy: An Essay on Interpretation*, trans. Dennis Savage. New Haven: Yale University Press.

Seligman, C. G. (1924) 'Anthropology and psychology: presidential address', *Journal of the Royal Anthropological Institute* 54: 13–46.

Tedlock, B. (1987a) 'Dreaming and dream research', in B. Tedlock (ed.) *Dreaming: Anthropological and Psychological Interpretations*. Cambridge: Cambridge University Press.

—— (1987b) 'Zuni and Quiche dream sharing and interpreting', in B. Tedlock (ed.) *Dreaming: Anthropological and Psychological Interpretations*. Cambridge: Cambridge University Press.

Tylor, E. B. (1871) *Primitive Culture: Researches into the Development of Mythology, Philosophy, Religion, Language, Art and Custom*. London: John Murray.

Ullman, M. D. and Zimmerman, N. (1989) *Working with Dreams*. Wellingborough: Aquarian Press.

7 Psychoanalysis, unconscious phantasy and interpretation

R. H. Hook

With his technical and intellectual equipment, the analyst undertakes to perform in a special way, and to encourage his patient towards a similar performance, namely to utilize consciousness (or the derivatives of unconscious processes) for the purpose of verbal thought, as distinct from action. This amounts to an undertaking to 'contain' the infantile aspects of the mind and only to communicate *about* them. This communication is the analyst's interpretative activity which will, in time, contribute to the patient's capacity for 'insight'. (Meltzer, 1967: xii)

The aim of this paper is to examine certain aspects of psychoanalytic interpretation and to suggest that psychoanalysis can best contribute to the understanding of culture and society through its understanding of mind.[1] What Meltzer is saying in the above quotation differs from more conventional, and especially from hermeneutic, ideas about interpretation. It may be useful to make a distinction between the 'process' of psychoanalysis and other aspects of psychoanalysis which might for convenience be summed up under 'content'. A comparable distinction was made by George Devereux (1967) between psychoanalysis as 'epistemology and methodology' and psychoanalysis as 'substantive data and theory'. The problem of defining precisely *what* content, if any, is specific to psychoanalysis will not be taken up here.

Meltzer is talking about psychoanalysis as process, the angle from which the question of interpretation will be approached, more specifically in regard to dream material.

George Devereux's clinical psychoanalytic work was done in the 1950s and early 1960s in the confident framework of classical psychoanalysis. There had already been challenges to an apparently established position: developments in the British Society had led to the so-called Controversial Discussions of the 1940s between Anna Freud and her group and those who followed Melanie Klein; Lacan's break with the Société Psychanalytique de Paris had occurred in 1953 but his views, formulated definitively at the Congress at Zurich in 1949, were little known, at least outside France, until the 1960s. Some, abandoning any attempt to find an empirical base, have sought other foundations: structuralist, Lacanian and hermeneutic interpretations compete with classical and related models. One is now confronted with psychoanalytic theories sufficiently diverse for a recent Presidential Address to the International Psychoanalytic Association to be entitled, 'One psychoanalysis or many?' (Wallerstein, 1988) and analysts themselves are concerned to find common ground, itself the theme of a recent international congress (Rome, 1989).

It is not necessary here to reflect upon the different philosophical assumptions, some of which concern the nature of psychoanalytic enquiry itself, which underlie these differences of opinion, though I agree with Elizabeth Spillius's comment that the empirical base of psychoanalysis lies in observation in the clinical setting (1988b: 223) and believe that the only way out of the present confusion of voices is to get back to this empirical base. In this essay several dreams are presented in order to comment on the nature of dreams and how they may be used in psychoanalytic interpretation; implications for the understanding of mind and its relation to culture will then be considered.

UNCONSCIOUS PHANTASY

The most significant development in Freud's theory lay in the introduction of the concepts of primary and secondary process and the identification of the significant role of phantasy, as it made possible a change of direction in psychoanalytic thinking away from a preoccupation with a model of the mind dealing with pressure, discharge and displacement of energy and the later model of conflict between psychic structures, towards more psychological notions like projection and projective identification, symbolic transformation and the theory of internal objects and object relations. Although an immediate application lay in the conclusion that trauma is not necessary for the later development of neurosis – it was similarly implicit that culture need not have arisen from an original parricide but could also be related to phantasy[2] – the significant consequence lay in a different conceptualisation of the mind, a more flexible model in which even the ego, defined as that part or aspect of the personality making contact with the external world, could be seen as developing out of a series of projections, introjections and identifications, making it largely an individual creation, in origin primitive and pre-verbal.

The concept of 'internal object' originated with Freud's notion of the super-ego, a mental institution deriving from the introjection of a parental figure or figures (though inevitably distorted by the child's own projections); this was a 'whole-object' introject. Melanie Klein extended and developed the concept of an introjected, hence internal, object and envisaged an earlier stage before things could be recognised and responded to as whole objects, a time when an infant is able to respond only to parts of its mother, her nipple or breast. These are introjected as 'part-objects', distorted also by the infant's own projections and no doubt having also an innate quality or component.

Melanie Klein held that when the infant takes in a satisfying feed it feels as though it has taken the good satisfying breast itself inside, and, conversely, when unsatisfied or hungry it not only feels empty, but as though there is a 'bad', that is, denying and frustrating, hence attacking and persecuting, breast inside. Primitive thinking (and by 'primitive' I intend 'rudimentary', in the sense where to speak of 'primitive man' would be to refer not to 'a native in a grass skirt' but to a unit of four or more dividing cells) is in terms of 'concrete' objects, not abstractions, and in terms of taking in or expelling, on the model of experienced bodily functions.[3] A very significant stage of development is reached when the infant first learns to respond to whole objects – mother as a whole person – and to become aware of the possibility of losing them. It was objected that an infant only months old could not have the neuronal equipment to support such functions; I think there is no way of settling definitively what an infant's mind is or is not capable of, but it has to be remembered that we are talking about the earliest stages of development of the mind, and mental activities must have appropriately rudimentary beginnings. It is because early phantasy is related to bodily processes and functions that psychoanalysts see what Lévi-Strauss refers to as *'le code psycho-organique'* as having a more fundamental role than other 'codes' (cf. Lévi-Strauss 1985: 243 ff.).

Internal phantasy objects, distorted by the infant's projective and introjective identifications, give rise, through symbolic transformations, to a whole internal world of phantasy objects in interaction with each other. An important distinction may then be seen to lie between an earlier classical Freudian theory employing only whole-object relationships and a newer way of conceptualising psychic activity in terms of transformations of, and relationships between, primitive part-objects as well as whole objects. Such a model of the mind, seen as developing out of introjected phantasy objects and part-objects, modified by an instinctual component and taken together with their subsequent symbolic transformations, offers a basis for the understanding of dream and other material from much later in life. The common and natural assimilation of myth to dream – natural because myth, like dream, rests, as Lévi-Strauss well demonstrates, on symbolic transformations – makes this newer conception of the mind of especial interest to the student of culture.

Following Susan Isaacs (1948), I take the concept phantasy to connote 'the primary content of unconscious mental process', a psychoanalytic 'technical' connotation which differs from the everyday use of the word. As this is a very different connotation from that of conscious fantasy it really requires a different word but, as one was not readily available and in view of the fact that the concept had been only gradually extended, Susan Isaacs resorted to the 'ph' spelling of phantasy (a usage authorised by the *Oxford English Dictionary*) to indicate that the extended meaning was the one intended. Unfortunately this extension has not been universally accepted though it is not always made clear whether it is only to the spelling that objection is taken or whether the extended meaning too is rejected.

What is needed here is a word, actually a more precise concept, to indicate an 'unknown', something occurring at an unconscious level; though obviously what is unconscious and unknown cannot be conceptualised otherwise than by inference from its known and observable consequences, a legitimate procedure and one adopted by theoretical physics. Wilfred Bion suggested that what is going on in the mind is unknown, indeed took it to be unknowable, comparing it with Kant's 'thing in itself'.[4] What *are* knowable are the transformations the 'thing-in-itself' undergoes. One such transformation (representation) is into unconscious phantasy.[5] Phantasies at least may become knowable: in dreams they may be observed directly and subsequently reported, though usually undergoing secondary revision in the process – phantasies still none the less. This is what makes phantasy so significant: there is no other product of the unconscious which can be so directly observed; hence dreams as 'the royal road to the unconscious' (Freud).

What I am proposing is a model of the mind in which quite diverse and relatively unknown mental operations can be transformed into phantasies which, though differing greatly among themselves, are each able to represent these operations or aspects of them; also that the content of the unconscious mind (i.e. mental events that are unconscious) can be transformed in an extremely volatile and flexible way into phantasy, while maintaining a basic stability, and one phantasy into another by symbolic transformation and substitution. Phantasies may be thought of as being some stable, some unstable and others existing only momentarily, if at all, their existence little more than potential, in this respect not unlike the molecules of chemistry.

I take the concept of 'defensive organisation'[6] to characterise the idea of something, in this case a defensive process, occurring unconsciously, which the patient may be in some way aware of and which can be learnt about through its being expressed in phantasies discoverable in dreams and other behaviour observable in analysis; 'internal objects' have a similar unconscious existence and are similarly discoverable.

DREAMS

These ideas may be illustrated in the analysis of several dreams, all of which show the overdetermination characteristic of dreams and phantasies. It is not necessary, for this purpose, to say much about the patient, Miss A, who had already been in analysis for some two to three years.

[1] I was in a church and it was your church, you were the priest or archbishop. I hadn't been to confession but I went inside just the same. When I got inside there was a service on, the altar was on the left and all the people were sitting in rows facing the altar. I didn't take communion. I was at the back of the church facing the other way, but it didn't seem to matter because I had a mirror.

A man with a moustache came up and touched me or took me by the hand; it was sexual and I felt embarrassed because we were in church. Then I was going for a holiday to somewhere on the coast. I didn't know where it was or how to get there but I had a picture of it, a beautiful inlet, and he was going to meet me there. It seemed a long way away but it was all right because I had a map and could find out how to get there.

The dream is clearly about the analyst and analysis, as is common enough, though usually more carefully disguised than in this dream. Analysis and analyst are idealised as church and archbishop or priest; though something is going on, Miss A does not participate but separates herself from it – she does not take communion or go to confession but sits at the back of the church, facing the wrong way. She was using, or rather *mis*using, the analysis in *her* way (but at some level recognising it to be the 'wrong' way), with her 'mirror' omnipotently watching what was going on in the analysis and turning it to her own (defensive) use. That she was misusing the analysis is not said lightly or in a pejorative way, it being taken for granted that patients misunderstand and misuse analyst and analysis for defensive purposes and that interpreting this is what analysis is largely about.

In the second part of the dream the analyst also figures, but now disguised as the 'man with a moustache', who seductively and embarrassingly touches A and arranges to meet her at a 'beautiful holiday inlet on the coast'. It is embarrassing to recognise sexual feelings towards the analyst, here reversed and attributed to the analyst himself, while the wish for a different kind of relationship with the analyst is also an expression of the defensive organisation. If for 'church' we read 'analysis', the explanation offered in the dream, 'because we were in church', reads, 'because we were in analysis'.

The seduction theme is maintained as the scene changes and the defensive organisation comes more clearly into force – with an escape to a 'beautiful holiday inlet', itself a representation of the defensive organisation. A different aspect of the defensive organisation is revealed in the following dream:

> [2] I was standing on a cliff and had a baby, the mother was standing behind me and wanting me to pick up the baby and look after it, but I said I would watch it and it would be all right. I was standing over it and then it started to crawl along near the edge of the cliff. Then it turned into my little dog and started to jump around, it jumped down on to a ledge and then it jumped again and into the water. I wanted to try to get down to rescue it from the heavy seas but it was too rough and I thought it was going to be drowned.

My interpretation was that the baby in the dream stood for the needy and dependent part of herself *and* for the understanding part of her mind which might co-operate in the analysis and of which she was only gradually becoming aware. The analyst (mother behind) was showing concern about the 'baby' and wanting her to pick it up and look after it, but instead, omnipotence took over: 'It'll be all right, *I'll* watch it', and it immediately crawled away into danger and over the edge of the cliff. The baby that might have been able to develop into something, with (analyst-) mother's help, turned into her little dog, the tricky, omnipotent part of herself that jumped around out of control and into danger.

In a third dream occurring some months later the defensive organisation appears as a demon, significantly in the top of a tree (standing for her mind):

> [3] I was walking with my dog and she was trying to get up into a tree and scratching and barking at something in the top of the tree, a demon or something, and it had taken something up there. I was hoping my dog would be able to get away because the demon was able to pull things up into the tree and I was terrified it would pull my dog up and it would be eaten or destroyed.

A's struggle towards a more satisfactory relationship with her internal objects was also shown in a dream which she said had consisted of three parts, but what she gave me was a confused mix of dream fragments and her own interpretations, of which only the third part was sufficiently coherent to report:

> [4] I was in Africa and I had a baby – but it wasn't quite like that; it wasn't really human, it was more a sort of animal and it might have been my dog. There was a boat with a lot of people in it, women, and someone threw it, my dog or my baby, and one of them was nursing it, and I didn't have it any more.

This dream seemed to show, rather poignantly, an attempt to create some-thing good, a good baby, despair of being able to achieve it and a sense of loss. It might have been a real baby (which she regretted not having had) but, and more significantly from the psychoanalytic point of view, it again represented a more positive and hopeful part of herself which she was trying to develop but over which she as yet had only a very insecure hold. What we see here is her constructive intention being taken over and perverted by the destructive defensive process: the baby becomes 'a sort of animal [or] it might have been my dog' – as it did in the earlier dream [2]. Significantly, she was very closely identified with her dog, to whom she gave a name reminiscent of herself.

Another dream a few months later further illustrated the continuing work with her internal objects; it was also in three parts, each of which revealed something of what had been happening in the analysis:

> [5] I was at a party or in a pub with Mr X and I was wanting to have a relationship with him. In the second part of the dream I had brought my parents to see him; they were very frail little old people with wizened faces, dried up skin and thin, weak spindly legs and they were sitting down waiting. In the third part, Mr X was telling me that I should use my special skills more or I would lose them. I think you might have been mixed up with Mr X.

A's wish to have an affair with Mr X ('mixed up with' the analyst) was complex and overdetermined: it contained at least the wish to be more comfortably placed and socially successful than her parents and an element of retaliating and triumphing over them (Mr X was seen as a conservative and socially successful politician who stood in marked contrast to her very radical and relatively poor parents); as well as identification with, and envy of, the analyst and his ability to understand and help. Envy is a significant factor in the establishment of defensive organisations and in blocking the path to more mature development. Her parents, in this dilapidated state, represented her still very damaged 'internal object' parents, though she was now beginning to feel some responsibility and was better able to see them not only as hateful, controlling, bigoted tyrants, but as the frail little old people in need of help and support that they probably were; accordingly, she was able in the dream to bring them along to get help too. Finally, she was noticing that she had indeed some valuable skills which she could lose unless she did something about developing them.

DREAMS, MYTHS AND CULTURE: PUBLIC AND PRIVATE PHANTASY

My impression is that, taken by themselves and on their manifest content alone, these dreams and their symbolism would not mean very much, nor could they be interpreted in terms of any fixed symbolism. Were a structural analysis of these dreams to be attempted, it is possible that what would emerge would be something that might be called the 'essential' dream and that it would turn out to be a phantasy representation of a defensive organisation or similar mental structure. Of necessity, I am able to see these dreams only in the context of an ongoing analysis of several years duration but in that context the dreams were a clarifying and useful commentary, showing what was going on in the patient's unconscious mind during this time and how the analysis was moving, information not otherwise available.

That dreams – or myths – should only reflect each other would seem to diminish their significance and raise a question as to whether anything so ultimately without meaning (*sc.* cause) occurs in nature? I was led to make this comment after reading a review of Lévi-Strauss's latest book, *La potière jalouse*: '[Lévi-Strauss's] more recent and, I think, more coherent view [is] that myths operate, as it were, in a hall of mirrors, but that they reflect only each other. This implies that myths – *and dreams* – are not mechanisms for communicating messages "*in a secret language*". They are best understood as modes of thinking, or perhaps, more precisely, reflection' (Kuper, 1989: 31, my emphasis).

The epithet 'secret' presumes a particular answer to the question of the nature of dream 'language', and implies an intent which is at best equivocal. It would be possible to formulate the apparent intent as a compromise: a compromise between the wish to communicate and the wish to conceal. Dreams, in Freud's view, represented a compromise between the expression of a drive or wish and its repression, in part concealing, in part revealing – a compromise we also see in myths. Paradoxical as it may seem, it is the wish to communicate that is unconscious, and that represents a drive towards reality and health, whereas the wish to conceal, not to know, is the more conscious, and serves the purpose of maintaining an unsatisfactory, but relatively stable, equilibrium, or status quo. Of course, to the extent that the patient voluntarily comes to analysis and communicates the dream apparently at least to be understood, whatever the defences erected against understanding, the communication is conscious in intent.

It can be agreed that it is as a mode of thinking that dreams are best understood, and are of most heuristic interest, the thinking being that of primary process in which wishes and anxieties and other contents and structures of the mind are represented in phantasies constructed and transformed according to the rules of a special kind of logic,[7] and through which the mind is able to communicate not only its content but the way in which it operates. What is suggested is that the above dreams show the mind to be in some way aware of, and able to communicate about, its own defensive organisation, employing different phantasies each of which is able to represent the whole constellation of phantasies through which in different forms the defensive organisation is expressed.

The other point that follows from the above line of reasoning is that dreams, or at least the dreams reported in analysis, are to be understood in the context of the ongoing analysis and may be seen as a communication to the analyst. To the objection that they are therefore 'compliant', or made under the influence of suggestion or to please the analyst, it has to be said that it would not have been possible for me to suggest the content of these dreams, or without them to have understood as well as I did what was going on. If compliant means an attempt to communicate with the analyst in terms which might be understood and interpreted by the analyst, then perhaps they are compliant. What the dreams also show is a wish and an ability both to know and not to know about, or not to accept, what at some level is recognised to be a barrier. Unconscious phantasy influences conscious attitudes and behaviour, and movement in unconscious phantasy systems, reflecting a shift in psychic equilibrium, mediates personality change and development. Dreams disclose phantasies operating at an unconscious level and may be the first indication of change in psychic equilibrium.

What I want to focus on here are the intrapsychic phantasy representations of defensive organisations and other 'structures' of the mind and the way in which they can be projected into the external world: I take this to be of significance also for the understanding of myth. A single structure of the mind, such as a defensive organisation, may be represented in dreams by many different phantasies, e.g., as an island, a house or building in which to take refuge, or, in other of its aspects, as an animal, a lion or a dog with aggressive or tricky features – all of these appeared in A's dreams at different times. One of the more revealing representations was that of the 'demon up in a tree' [3], showing that, though not necessarily consciously, she knew of it and what it was doing to her mind. The demon in the top of the tree represented something going on in the 'top' part of her, her mind, that caught things up and complicated them in a destructive way, making them unavailable for understanding and use; similarly the little dog itself, as a 'tricky', 'running away', 'getting into danger' little dog, stood for the defensive organisation and showed how it operated.

The above interpretations of these dreams may be taken to illustrate contemporary psychoanalytic understanding and use of symbolism. Symbols are very fluid constructions, individual, specific and idiosyncratic, though following generally applicable principles of a logical kind, illustrated, for example, in the various symbolic representations of 'container' and 'contained'.[8] Were they not in accord with some such principles, symbols would not be understandable and would be useless for purposes of communication, including intrapsychic communication. What the patient is symbolising in the case reported is her own behaviour in avoiding recognising and coming to terms with her failures and disappointments. Interpretation takes the form, not so much of saying 'This is what the dream, or the phantasies, mean', as of using the information contained in and communicated through the dream to show the analysand not only how he or she sees and uses analyst and analysis, but also how this defensive behaviour is expressed in daily life; the problems this created being what brought the patient to analysis in the first place.

I now return to the concept of defensive organisation as a 'structure' of the mind and try to show how projections of this kind of structure might be significant for culture. Herbert Rosenfeld, who worked with the concept of narcissistic organisation in the early 1960s, noted that 'when a patient of this kind makes progress in the analysis and wants to change he dreams of being attacked by members of the Mafia or adolescent delinquents' (Rosenfeld, 1971: 174) – an obvious personification, though one deriving from the dream phantasies of patients in analysis. When an individual dreams of, say, a Mafia, he or she takes something from the external world to characterise and represent an aspect of internal reality, thereby linking unconscious phantasy and the external world. When I was trying to show my patient how she had internalised and identified with a party organiser's arrogant and obsessional control of his particular political group, expelling any who weakened, deviated or otherwise failed, she added spontaneously, 'The Central Committee of the Communist Party!' This political organisation corresponded to Miss A's own defensive phantasy system in that it represented an omnipotent intolerance of any weakness or failure.

Here the defensive system finds reinforcement in identification with an already existing social institution but, in the absence of any such institution, it may be possible by political or other activity to set one up. The mind then recreates its own image and replicates itself externally. Mythical and other ritual and belief systems and institutions may function in this way, facilitating shared identifications. This being so, may we not then begin to see some explanation for those transformations of myth which are central to Lévi-Strauss's thinking? They correspond to varied projections of internal structures and are established in mutually shared projective identifications.

Examples have been given of identification with the Mafia and with the Central Committee of the Communist Party, but history offers many examples of institutions similarly fitting presumed unconscious needs. The Calvinist doctrine of predestination suggests omnipotent identification with 'the Will of God': the 'Elect' impose their will on others, as did the Holy Office of the

Inquisition and the Committee of Public Safety of the French Revolution, with extreme cruelty, claiming it to be the 'Will of God', for the 'Good of the Community', for the 'Protection' of the Revolution, or 'Truth', or whatever happened to be the context at the time.[9]

To summarise, if internal phantasy can be projected into existing systems in the external world or if suitable systems can be created and external reality so made to conform to, or reflect, internal phantasy, the internal phantasy system is felt to be confirmed by external reality and is accordingly reinforced: a system of projective and introjective identification (with reprojection and reintrojection and seeming to carry its own validation within itself) is then set up and external organisation ('public' fantasy) reflects or mirrors internal organisation ('private' phantasy) in a reciprocal and mutually reinforcing relationship.

STRUCTURE OF MIND

It is doubtful whether the structure of the mind could be understood at all were it not for one striking characteristic of the mind: its capacity to project itself and its structure. It is this capacity, more specifically the mechanism of projective identification as it bears on the analyst's counter-transference, that makes psychoanalysis possible and distinguishes it from all other therapies.[10]

Devereux's great contribution to the analysis of art was to point out that the pivotal feature of art, upon which the very possibility of art depends, is that the work of art replicates in its own structure the structure of the mind.[11] In 'The mind and the mind's image of itself', Richard Wollheim, to illustrate the way in which the mind is aware of its internal objects, takes as example the way in which the mind uses internal figures, both awake and in dreams, and compares this with the way in which a novelist or playwright invents and uses characters: to speak his words and to express his thoughts (Wollheim, 1969: 211). Freud made a similar observation: 'The projected creations of primitive men resemble the personifications constructed by creative writers; for the latter externalize in the form of separate individuals the opposing instinctual impulses struggling within them' (Freud, 1913: 65n).

What is psychoanalysis? Is it many, or is it one? If there were to be many psychoanalyses it would follow that the respects in which they differed could not be essential to psychoanalysis but only that respect in which they corresponded: if aX, aY and aZ are three prospective candidates for psychoanalytic status, it cannot be X, Y or Z that is psychoanalysis but only that which they have in common, a. This a should be a specific and identifiable process,[12] whereas it is likely that X, Y and Z will be found to be different theories about mind, or 'content'.

Process implies and requires structure. Freud discovered the psycho-analytic process and postulated several possible 'structures' – working models of the mind: the 'topographical' theory, the 'structural' theory and so on, generally referred to as his metapsychology. It was the process that Freud discovered that is central to psychoanalysis: transference and the interpretation of transference, dependent upon the 'setting' which psycho-analysis creates and which is essential to it. Equally important for practice is the analyst's counter-transference, and what the analyst is able to per-ceive of the effects on him or her of the patient's transference: this is the basis on which interpretations are constructed.

Psychoanalytic understanding and interpretation imply a model of the mind. That adopted here is based on phantasy as 'the primary content of unconscious mental activity' and a concept of transformations: an 'unknown' becoming known through transformation into phantasy, the mind thereby also becoming, to a degree, aware of itself and the way in which it operates.

NOTES

1 This is a condensed version of a paper presented at the Paris colloquium; limitations of space make it impossible to present all the clinical material upon which my understanding of these dreams and hence my interpretations are based.

2 'Accordingly the mere hostile *impulse* against the father, the mere existence of a wishful *phantasy* of killing and devouring him, would have been enough to produce the moral reaction that created totemism and taboo' (Freud, 1913: 159–60).

3 Matte-Blanco introduced a new dimension into the discussion of the concepts of internal and external as applied to the mind, of internal world, internal objects and thinking in terms of 'concrete' objects (1988: 124 ff., *passim*). In thinking about the mind we constantly resort to physical metaphors, especially of the body and of space.

4 'Ding an sich' presents considerable philosophic difficulties and it is possible that in his later work Kant abandoned the concept. See Kemp Smith 1930: 204–5, *passim*.

5 My comment. I am not clear whether this view was held by Bion, either explicitly or implicitly, though I suspect he would not have disagreed. There is reason to think that what limits our knowing is not that the basic functions of the mind as such are unknowable but our incapacity so far to formulate or conceptualise them. Although I refer to basic, and unconscious, mental func-tions, I ignore for the purposes of this discussion the question of relationship to physical (brain) process and treat mind as equally real.

6 When confronted with a painful situation such as the recognition of failure, disappointment and loss, or the need to accept suffering, the mind, instead of accepting the reality, may attempt evasion by deploying primitive defence mechanisms, typically splitting, manic denial, projection and projective

126   *The analysis of dreams*

identification, leading to narcissistic omnipotence, and this may occur in such a way as to result in the formation of a stable, organised system of defences with recognisable consequences for personality development, a 'defensive organisation', also referred to in the literature as 'narcissistic' or 'pathological' organisation. (See further, Rosenfeld, 1965, 1971, 1987; Spillius, 1983, 1988a; O'Shaughnessy, 1981; Steiner, 1987, 1990).

7 For a fuller discussion of primary process logic, phantasy and symbol formation, see Hook, 1979; Matte-Blanco, 1988: 174, *passim*.

8 I am indebted to R. T. Martin, lately Professor of Psychology at the University of New South Wales, for valuable comment on an earlier draft of this paper, especially on the psychoanalytic use of dream symbols.

9 'In projective identification parts of the self and internal objects are split off and projected into the external object, which then becomes possessed by, controlled and identified with the projected parts' (Segal, 1964: 27).

10 See Jaques, 1955: 480 ff.

11 'The problem is entirely one of recognizing the transformation of psychic content into art or the artistic representation of psychic mechanisms. In effect, independently of what the mind is able to contemplate, imitate or create, what it inevitably does is to reproduce itself' (Devereux, 1975: 55, my translation).

12 'One might say that the value of the analytical process derives from the degree to which it is determined by the structure of the mind. The link is of course the "transference" and the "counter-transference", unconscious and infantile functions of the minds of patient and analyst' (Meltzer, 1967: xi–xii).

BIBLIOGRAPHY

Bion, W. R. (1962) *Learning from Experience*. London: Heinemann.
—— (1963) *Elements of Psycho-Analysis*. London: Heinemann.
—— (1965) *Transformations: Change from Learning to Growth*. London: Heinemann.
—— (1970) *Attention and Interpretation: A Scientific Approach to Insight in Psycho-Analysis and Groups*. London: Tavistock.
Devereux, G. (1967) *From Anxiety to Method in the Behavioral Sciences*. The Hague: Mouton.
—— (1975) *Tragedie et Poesie Grecques: Etudes Ethnopsychanalytiques*. Paris: Flammarion.
Freud, S. (1913) *Totem and Taboo, S.E.* 13: 1–162.
Hook, R. H. (1979) 'Phantasy and symbol: a psychoanalytic point of view', in R. H. Hook (ed.) *Fantasy and Symbol: Studies in Anthropological Interpretation*. London and New York: Academic Press.
Isaacs, S. (1948) 'The nature and function of phantasy', *International Journal of Psycho-Analysis* 29: 73–9. Reprinted in P. King and R. Steiner (eds) *The Freud–Klein Controversies 1941–45*. London: Routledge, 1991.
Jaques, E. (1955) 'Social systems as defence against persecutory and depressive anxiety: a contribution to the psycho-analytical study of social processes', in M. Klein, P. Heimann and R. Money-Kyrle (eds) *New Directions in Psycho-Analysis*. London: Tavistock.
Kemp Smith, N. (1930) *A Commentary to Kant's 'Critique of Pure Reason'*. London: Macmillan.
Kuper, A. (1989) 'Symbols in myths and dreams: Freud v. Lévi-Strauss', *Encounter* March: 26–31.

Lévi-Strauss, C. (1985) *La potière jalouse*. Paris: Librairie Plon.
Matte-Blanco, I. (1988) *Thinking, Feeling, and Being: Clinical Reflections on the Fundamental Antinomy of Human Beings and World*. London and New York: Routledge.
Meltzer, D. (1967) *The Psycho-Analytical Process*. Perthshire: Clunie, reprinted 1979.
O'Shaughnessy, E. (1981) 'A clinical study of a defensive organization', *International Journal of Psycho-Analysis* 62: 359–69; also in E. B. Spillius (ed.) 1988a.
Rosenfeld, H. A. (1965) 'On the psychopathology of narcissism: a clinical approach', in *Psychotic States: A Psychoanalytical Approach*. London: Hogarth.
—— (1971) 'A clinical approach to the psychoanalytic theory of the life and death instincts', *International Journal of Psycho-Analysis* 52: 169–78; also in E. B. Spillius (ed.) 1988a.
—— (1987) *Impasse and Interpretation: Therapeutic and Anti-Therapeutic Factors*. London: Tavistock.
Segal, H. (1964) *Introduction to the Work of Melanie Klein*. London: Hogarth, rev. edn, 1973.
Spillius, E. B. (1983) 'Some developments from the work of Melanie Klein', *International Journal of Psycho-Analysis* 64: 321–2.
—— (ed.) (1988a) *Melanie Klein Today: Developments in Theory and Practice*, Vol. 1, *Mainly Theory*. London and New York: Routledge.
—— (ed.) (1988b) *Melanie Klein Today: Developments in Theory and Practice*, Vol. 2, *Mainly Practice*. London and New York: Routledge.
Steiner, J. (1987) 'The interplay between pathological organizations and the paranoid-schizoid and depressive positions', *International Journal of Psycho-Analysis* 68: 69–80.
—— (1990) 'Pathological organizations as obstacles to mourning: the role of unbearable guilt', *International Journal of Psycho-Analysis* 71: 87–94.
Wallerstein, R. S. (1988) 'One psychoanalysis or many?', *International Journal of Psycho-Analysis* 69: 5–21.
Wollheim, R. (1969) 'The mind and the mind's image of itself', *International Journal of Psycho-Analysis* 50: 209–20.

Part III
The Lacanian perspective

8 Gendered persons
Dialogues between anthropology and psychoanalysis

Henrietta Moore

Issues of human identity, intention and agency have always engaged the attention of philosophers. In recent years, they have become the focus of anthropological enquiry. One result of this has been an explosion of interest in indigenous concepts of person and self. What is interesting about this research is that although it has developed contemporaneously with the anthropology of gender there has been little attempt to bring these two fields of enquiry together. Indigenous concepts of the person and the self are presented, most often, as gender neutral, but on closer examination it is clear that the implicit model for the person in much ethnographic writing is, in fact, an adult male.[1] The apparent resistance to joining these two domains of enquiry is curious for a number of reasons. Firstly, anthropologists have long recognised that there are many instances in which women and men are thought to be different sorts of person as a consequence of their different gender identities. Secondly, an explicit concern in much anthropological writing on the person with the boundaries and physical constitution of the person, and with the associated questions of agency and intention, raises immediate questions about the relationship between personal identity and embodiment. One such link is evident, for example, in the case of procreation beliefs, where ideas about the physical make-up of the body are closely connected both to ideas about the nature of the person and to ideas about gender. Thirdly, the demarcation of the anthropology of the person/self from the anthropology of gender seems particularly curious given the fact that psychoanalysis provides western culture with a model of the acquisition of human subjectivity and identity which is crucially dependent on sexual difference.[2] The subject of psychoanalysis is always a sexed subject.

ANTHROPOLOGY AND ITS THEORIES OF PERSON AND SELF

Anthropologists have never assumed that the western concept of the person is universal, and, almost uniquely among academic disciplines, they have

132 *The Lacanian perspective*

the data to show that this is the case. However, in the face of recent post-structuralist and deconstructionist critiques of the unified, rational subject of western humanist discourse, anthropologists have remained perversely silent; they have scarcely contributed to the debate at all.

This silence is hard to interpret. There are those who would point to the hostility displayed towards post-structuralist and deconstructionist approaches in the discipline. The strange fact of the matter is that, while most anthropologists are strongly social constructionist and, less often, culturally relativist in their thinking, they have a firm allegiance to the empirical nature of ethnographic facts. The result is a fruitful, but uneasy tension between social constructionism and empiricism.

The ambivalent relations between empiricism and social constructionism apparent in anthropological writing and theorising are partly the product of the political liberalism which historically has informed much anthropological thinking. This is not to say that all anthropologists are liberals – such a statement would patently be false – but rather that anthropology has maintained a commitment to the sovereign nature of individuals, to the coherence and rationality of their beliefs, values and lifeways, and to their right to self-determination. In this context, it is quite unsurprising that anthropology – or rather a significant number of its practitioners – should be resistant to post-structuralist and deconstructionist attempts to undermine the Cartesian *cogito*, the 'I' who authors experience of self and of the world, and who is also the essence at the core of identity. This resistance should be understood from at least two perspectives. Firstly, there is the understandable reluctance, equally evident in the writings of many feminist theorists (e.g., Tress, 1988; Flax, 1987), to relinquish the idea that all persons are rational, unified individuals, in favour of a view of the subject and of subjectivity which stresses its shifting, imaginary and conflicting nature. This latter view, while absolutely harmless for the average western male academic, could so easily become a pathological characterisation of others. Secondly, there is the question of the anthropologists themselves and of their role in the production of anthropological knowledge. Anthropologists have historically based their knowledge of another culture on their experience of that culture: an experience which is both authentic and unique. Post-structuralist and deconstructionist readings of the subject emphasise that the 'I' does not author experience, that there is no singular essence at the core of each individual which makes them what they are and which guarantees the authenticity of their knowledge of self and of the world. It is clear from both these perspectives that post-structuralist and deconstructionist accounts of the subject would appear to threaten the anthropological project.

Appropriately enough, however, this threat is more apparent than real. This is evident if we turn to examine anthropological findings and arguments about the person and the self cross-culturally. Anthropological work on the self, known variously as indigenous psychology, ethnopsychology and cultural psychology, embodies many different approaches and philosophical positions. Such differences frequently oscillate around questions of universality. A large body of work draws on the writings of Irving Hallowell (1971) and G. H. Mead (1934). In such work, the capacity for self-awareness, the ability to distinguish self from other (self-identity) and the apprehension of self-continuity are thought to be essential for basic human and cultural functioning. In short, they are considered as universal attributes of the self. These universal attributes, however, do not imply anything about the local views of the self which will be prevalent in any particular culture. Many anthropologists have been very specific about the fact that these universal attributes underpin all local conceptions, but that they are not to be confused with a western concept of the self. The western concept of the self is simply another local model.

Anthropologists remain very divided over the degree to which local, culturally constructed, models of the self can be seen to be constitutive of psychological processes per se. The controversy rumbles on: some arguing that processes such as memory do not make much sense outside the culturally constructed concepts of memory and the way in which those concepts determine the experience of memory, while others insist that memory is a function that operates and/or exists independently of the way in which it might be conceptualised in specific contexts.

Less controversial is the anthropological recognition that indigenous concepts of the self vary in the way in which they conceptualise the relationship between self and non-self, the degree to which mind (if it exists at all) is separated from body, and the manner in which agency and motivation are conceptualised as arising internally or externally to the self. More importantly, perhaps, concepts like the unconscious are seen to be highly culturally specific, as are ideas about the bounded and unitary nature of the self. These kinds of arguments in anthropology are not only supported by cross-cultural analysis, but they have gained credibility through their comparison with historical data on the changing nature of western concepts of the self over time. Anthropology's slow recognition of variability in western discourses, on this and other matters, has been due, by and large, to the discipline's need for a stable set of concepts, categories and discourses through which to view other cultures. However, the acknowledgement of variability does not entirely dispose of the unease which many anthropologists feel regarding social constructionist arguments. In other words, just because people do not speak of having an unconscious and do not discursively or practically recognise the existence and functioning of the unconsciousness does not mean that they do not have an unconscious or that unconscious processes do not influence their developmental psychology.

Nominalism may be a perennial problem in anthropology, but it seems equally implausible to suggest that discourses and discursive practices are not constitutive of experience. It seems clear that, since all psychic and developmental processes are clearly relational, then the nature of the relationship between self and other(s), and the matrix of social relations and symbolic systems within which that relationship is conducted, must play a key role in the development of the self and of subjectivity. It seems pertinent, therefore, that in many cultures people do not believe that selves and persons are bounded and they do not think that embodiment is the essence of identity.

Germaine Dieterlen argued in the 1940s that the Dogon believe that a person remains in a permanent relation with other persons, and with aspects of the natural world, in such a way that these human and non-human elements are constitutive of the person (Dieterlen, 1941). Similar arguments, drawing on Mauss, have been made, of course, for a number of African societies (e.g., Lienhardt, 1985). Also in the 1940s, Maurice Leenhardt argued that the Canaque of New Caledonia regard the person as being connected to other persons, both human and non-human, material and non-material. What is more they conceive the body as a temporary locus, and not as the source of individual identity (Leenhardt, 1979 [1947]). Anne Strauss's work on the Cheyenne emphasises that the Cheyenne self participates in, and therefore cannot be defined by contrast with, other Cheyenne selves. Furthermore, the concept of person extends beyond human beings to include other non-human persons. For the Cheyenne, relationships with non-human persons are crucial for the development of the self. The categorical identification between persons and human beings on which western social science and many other indigenous western discourses are based is ruptured (Strauss, 1982: 124–5). Similarly, the relationship between self, self-identity and experience has been brought into question by a number of writers. Jean Smith has suggested that, for the Maori, it was generally not the self which encompassed experience, but experience which encompassed the self. According to Smith (1981: 152), the Maori individual was conceived of as being made up of various independent organs of experience, and these organs each reacted to external stimuli independently of the self. Thus the self was not viewed as controlling experience, and an individual's experience was not felt to be integral to the self.

This brief review of some indigenous theories of the person and the self raises two very interesting points. The first concerns the extent to which persons who are not thought to be separate from other persons (both human and non-human) can be conceived of as individuals. In an earlier period in anthropology, it was fashionable to follow Mauss in arguing that the self was a social product, and that in primitive societies it was relatively undifferentiated. The individual was seen as a modern construct, and individualism was thought to be a feature of modern societies. Mauss himself was careful not to slip into a crude evolutionism, but much anthropological writing remains fascinated by the problem of individualism, and by the question of whether or not it is, in some sense, the product of modern living. This view, in some attenuated form, could be said to underlie Dumont's (1970) writings on India. However, a slightly different strand of anthropological thinking has sought to emphasise that, while persons in some societies might be thought of as inseparable from other persons, this does not mean that individuals do not exist or that people's actions are not evaluated in terms of an individual life trajectory or career. Meyer Fortes (1973) made this sort of argument for the Tallensi.[3] What is interesting about this debate in anthropology is that it betrays an anxiety about whether persons who are not separate from other persons or who are defined in relation to significant others can be said to have the appropriate capacities for agency and intention. The western folk model that underpins anthropological theorising is, in fact, much indebted to psychoanalysis and therefore it has difficulty in conceiving that an adult person who is not separate from other persons could be capable of agency and intention. Hence the necessity to insist that the Tallensi are individuals, even if they are bound into a 'web of kinship' in such a way that they do not conceive of themselves as separate persons.

The second point concerns the relationship between identity, self-identity and physical embodiment. Once again, the western folk model underlying anthropological theorising does not accommodate itself easily to the suggestion that the body is not always the source and locus of identity, and that the interior self is not necessarily the source or locus of intention or agency. The idea of persons as divisible, partible and unbounded has now gained a certain acceptance in the discipline (see, for example, Marriott, 1976; Strathern, 1988), but there is still considerable resistance to any suggestion that the body might not be the source of identity, or that experience (both of self and of the world) is not always possessed by or located in an interior self.

The point which emerges then from a review of anthropological writings on indigenous concepts of the person and the self is that ethnographic data appear to support the post-structuralist and deconstructionist critique of the Cartesian *cogito*. It is quite clear that the western transcendental subject and the western concept of the person are far from universal. It is evident also that, while self-awareness may be a universal human attribute, this is not the same thing as saying that everyone has a phenomenological and/or conceptual category of the self which corresponds to the western concept of the self. The variation which exists in the understanding, definition and experience of the self, and in the self's relations with other selves and with the world does not make the individuals concerned incapable of agency or intention. The anxieties of feminists and anthropologists that post-structuralist views of the subject might prove pathologising may very well be justified politically, but they are not so easy to justify from a theoretical point of view. It would seem that the only reason why alternative concepts of the person and self appear so threatening is that they challenge western folk models of the person/self, and they thus undermine knowledge claims based on subject–object dualisms and the transcendental nature of the knowing subject.

However, cross-cultural variability is not the only issue. A more serious difficulty is raised by the existence of multiple models and/or discourses within cultures, societies, groups or sets of people. Anthropologists have only recently begun to discuss and to document the existence of multiple models, and to look at the variation which exists within cultures as well as between them. This development, which has clear origins in the rise of feminist and Marxist anthropology, has forced a certain re-evaluation of the concept of culture. The current emphasis on culture as a competing, con-tested and conflicting domain of meanings has provided the opportunity for an investigation of multiple models. The result is that anthropologists are more aware than ever of the fact that it is impossible to speak of a particular culture as having one model of the person or one conception of the self. What seems evident is that, although multiple discourses exist, some dis-courses are dominant over others and some are appropriate only to specific contexts. In the case of discourses on the person and the self, what appear as dominant models may actually turn out to be relatively divorced from everyday life and experience.

For example, the dominant model of the person/self in western Europe could be said to be one which characterises the individual as rational, autonomous and unitary. This individual is the author of their own experi-ence and of their knowledge of the world, and their existence is enshrined in post-Enlightenment philosophy, in political theory and in legislation. However, this model of the person/self, which would be accessible through anthropological analysis, has a very complex relationship with the every-day experiences and practices of women and men in Europe. Many people, I would venture to suggest, have occasions when they find it extremely difficult to conceive of themselves as rational, autonomous and unitary. Western European culture has evolved a number of ways, many of them connected to religious belief, to deal with the fact that individuals do not necessarily experience themselves as the authors of their own experience and of their knowledge of the world. As a result, many alternative discourses on the person/self exist, some of them more formalised than others, some of them developed in explicit contradistinction to the dominant model. The task for anthropologists is to investigate how their own popular discourses or folk models inform the academic discourses which they have at their disposal, and to examine how dominant models relate to alternative popular discourses in the societies they study.

GENDER AND IDENTITY[4]

This task is a particularly important one when it comes to the anthropological study of gender because in many cases, including western cultures, concepts of the person and the self are connected to models for explaining gender difference. This point needs emphasis because of the way in which it is assumed in much anthropological writing that concepts of the person and the self are gender neutral. This assumption seems to be based on the premise that the person and the self are ontologically prior to gender identity, that is, to the gendered self.

This interesting view contains a number of further premises. One is the idea common in western social science and philosophy that the person is to be understood as an entity that has ontological priority over the various roles and activities through which it engages in social practices and comes to have social meaning and significance. This idea logically presupposes an essence at the core of the person which exists prior to the person's insertion into a social matrix and which is fixed over time. Within philosophical discourse, the question of what constitutes personal identity focuses on the question of what establishes the continuity or self-identity of the person over time. It would not be appropriate to enter into these debates here, but, in terms of anthropological discourse, it seems quite clear that the most important characteristic of the person over time, and the one which constitutes its identity, is the fact of physical embodiment. This assumption, which is very prevalent in anthropological writing and which is often implicit rather than explicit, is clearly part of a western discourse, rather than a natural fact of human existence. The earlier review of indigenous concepts of the person and the self cast doubt on the assumption that persons are necessarily conceived of as bounded entities with fixed essences, and it questioned the assumption that the body is always the source and locus of identity. This does not mean, of course, that the fact of embodiment is unimportant, but it does mean that it cannot be unproblematically taken as the logical or defining feature of the person or of personal identity through time. Attributes of personhood, such as the continuity and coherence of the person through time, are socially and culturally established, they are not merely given in the physical fact of embodiment. Self-identity is thus something that has to be established socially through a set of discourses which are both discursive and practical. These discourses establish the grounds for identity, and the framework(s) within which identity becomes intelligible.

As Judith Butler has pointed out in her brilliant discussion of these arguments, it is clear that, within western cultural discourses, ideas about gender identity form a crucial part of the framework within which self-identity becomes intelligible (1990: 16–17). This is very much as we should expect, given that psychoanalytic discourse provides us with a model for the acquisition of human identity and subjectivity which is crucially dependent on binary sexual difference. While certain philosophical discourses may give ontological primacy to the person and the self *vis-à-vis* gender identity, it is quite clear that in psychoanalytic and popular discourse the person and the self are not considered as gender neutral. When discourses on the person and the self are approached via discourses on gender, the ontological status of gender in western discourse becomes apparent. Gender identity is manifestly assumed to be the essence at the core of personal identity in many western discourses. Much contemporary feminist theory, for example, employs such an assumption about the ontological status of gender, as is evident in the use of the all important verb 'to be'. The claim 'to be' a woman has recently become politically and theoretically problematic in feminist discourse, but in many other popular discourses it remains quite unproblematic.

The ontological status of gender in terms of western discourses on the person and the self is reinforced by the assumption that physical embodiment is the logical and defining feature of the person and of personal identity through time. The elision between gender identity and physical embodiment accounts for the extraordinary emphasis in western discourse on the sexually differentiated nature of the human body. The argument that the binary characterisation of gender is self-evident because there are two clearly differentiated and natural categories of the body provides the basis for the grounding of gender differences in the biologically given facts of sex. Feminist theory in the social sciences has striven, in the last twenty years, to separate sex from gender, in order to demonstrate that gender is a social construction, and is not given in biology or in nature. It is interesting that one very common response to this feminist strategy has been the simple riposte that women and men have biological functions and that it is impossible to escape the fact that human societies need to reproduce. What is curious about this riposte is that it is an extraordinarily weak one, but it is considered by those who reproduce it to be particularly strong. It appears strong, of course, because it is securely grounded within the dominant, naturalised and self-evident discourse regarding gender identity and embodiment. Yanagisako and Collier (1987) have recently pointed out that, although the feminist strategy of separating sex from gender appears to challenge dominant western models, it actually reproduces the very same assumptions on which those models are based. Paradoxically, the separation of sex from gender reinforces the idea that there are two clearly differentiated and natural categories of the body. While gender is not determined by sex, it is seen as a cultural mechanism for managing the fact of sexual difference. The result is that, while the meanings attributed to women and men in any culture may be variable, there is never any doubt that gender is on the body, and the evidence for this is the very fact of sexual differentiation.

The idea that gender is on the body, and that gender has an ontological status which defines the parameters within which personal identity becomes intelligible, cannot be considered, of course, to be universally applicable. If we turn to look at non-western views of gender difference and the role such difference plays in framing or determining personal identity, we see that gender is often held to have an ontological status, but that its relationship to the question of embodiment is thought to be rather different. Deborah Gewertz discusses Tchambuli views of gender difference, embodiment and personal identity. She observes that her participation in meetings in the men's house gave rise to a situation where she herself was characterised as 'probably not a woman at all, but a strange creature who grew male genitals upon donning trousers' (1984: 618). Her husband was thought to be a feminised male and her daughter was considered to have been purchased from a stranger who needed money. This redefinition did not affect Gewertz's status as an individual, but it did effectively render her a non-person. To be a person among the Tchambuli is to be a member of a patriclan, and through the possession of certain names, inherited both from the person's patrilineal ancestors and from his or her father's affines, to become the repository of both patrilineal and matrilineal relationships. The definition of personhood among the Tchambuli is therefore one based on the embodiment of these relationships. As an hermaphroditic woman, Gewertz was effectively self-contained, with neither affines nor kin. She was unable to produce children whose kin would have to be compensated, and thus she was a non-person (Gewertz, 1984: 619).

There are several interesting points to be made about the situation Gewertz describes. Firstly, the Tchambuli conception of the relationship between gender and embodiment is somewhat different from that which pertains under the so-called western model, although there are also some similarities. Gender is certainly located in the body in some sense, because the performance of male activities gives rise to the presumption that this involves the acquisition of male genitals. The issue here is not, of course, whether the Tchambuli do or do not think that Gewertz really acquired male genitals. What is important is that gender identity is given as much by the performance of appropriate activities, as it is by the possession of the appropriate genitalia. Secondly, there is the question of whether gender identity can be seen as the essence at the core of personal identity. In one sense, this would certainly seem to be the case because becoming classed as an hermaphrodite apparently rendered Gewertz a non-person. However, the crucial point here is not that she was of indeterminate gender, but that being sexually complete made her incapable of social reproduction, the production of persons being the vehicle for the reproduction of social relationships. This is connected to a third point about what guarantees the identity or self-identity of a person over time. In this example, it seems that identity is guaranteed by a matrix of social relationships, rather than by anything which might be deemed an essential attribute of the individual.

Recent ethnography has produced evidence of a number of cases where it is the performance of particular kinds of activities or tasks which guarantees gender identity rather than simply the possession of the appropriate genitalia. This is the argument, for example, that Harriet Whitehead (1981) has made for the Berdache of North America, and that Jane Atkinson (1990) makes for the Wana of Indonesia. These findings stress the importance given in many indigenous models to performance in the determination of gender identity rather than to arguments about essential attributes. In such models, physical characteristics are the sign or effect of sexual difference rather than the cause of gender identity. It is for this reason that if you are a woman who behaves like a man then you must grow a penis (Gewertz, 1984: 619; Atkinson, 1990: 88–93). In fact, of course, a certain discourse on the relationship between performance or social enactment and gender identity exists in western cultures. It is just that this discourse is, by and large, subordinate to the dominant discourse which stresses the essential and embodied nature of gender identity.

There are a number of other non-western views of gender difference that stress the ontological status of gender, but do so in a way which questions the relationship between gender and embodiment established in western discourse. A number of indigenous procreation beliefs and anatomical theories involve ideas about gendered substances and the multiply gendered nature of human bodies. One familiar set of ideas concerns the flesh and bone kinship discussed by Lévi-Strauss (Lévi-Strauss, 1969). Models of this kind stress the ontological status of gender, but they also stress that gender differences exist within bodies rather than simply or solely between them. Thus persons are multiply gendered, and a model which stresses that the body can be divided into two naturally occurring and mutually exclusive categories cannot hope to explain the relationship between gender and embodiment which these theories propose. Anna Meigs discusses gender identity and embodiment among the Hua of the New Guinea Highlands where the determination of gender is a complex and multiple process and does not depend on external genitalia alone. The Hua classify gender on the basis of whether or not persons contain in their bodies greater or lesser amounts of certain substances (menstrual blood, parturitional fluids, vaginal secretions) classed as female. Women lose these fluids as they get older and hence they become masculinised. Men, on the other hand, absorb more of these fluids over time, through sex, eating and casual contact, and they become feminised as they age (Meigs, 1990: 108–11). Among the Hua, female/male is not a singular and simple opposition. Gender may be in the body, but it exists within bodies as well as between them, and it has no ontological status, nor can it be said to be the fixed essence at the core of personal identity.

Ethnographic examples like the above reinforce the point that anthropological findings question a number of assumptions which are implicit in dominant western discourses on the relationship between personhood, gender identity and embodiment. In particular, anthropological data question the notion of a single, undisputed and fixed gender at the core of the person. One immediate difficulty with ethnographic material on such issues as personhood and gender identity is that it is unclear what the relationship might be between cultural theories about sexual substances, for example, and the actual experience of being a gendered individual in Hua society. There is a potential discrepancy between a discourse or set of discourses which are culturally available and the individual experience, interpretation and understanding of those discourses. However, as discussed by a number of theorists, there is no meaning to being a gendered self outside the set of culturally available discourses within which being a gendered self finds meaning. This does not mean, of course, that individuals are not able to resist or disagree with cultural discourses. They clearly are able to do this. But even moments of resistance are moments of compliance, and discourses which conflict are often constituted in contradistinction to each other. It therefore follows that the experience of being a gendered self in a context where gender differences are thought to lie as much within bodies as between them, and where aspects of one's gender identity are thought to be fluid and changeable is likely to be significantly different from the experience of being a gendered self in a context which stresses the fixed and mutually exclusive nature of binary gender categories. It seems quite implausible to suggest that psychic development is not affected by these very different ideas about the relationship of individuals to themselves, to others and to their world. This seems crucially important given the fact that the development of self-awareness involves relations with others (i.e., intersubjectivity), as well as language. Without these two things the development of self-awareness would be impossible. The development of the self and of self-awareness is thus both discursively and practically produced. The particular force of cultural discourses, of course, is that they have material affects, that they are practically or performatively, as well as discursively, maintained (Bourdieu, 1976, 1990). Consequently, theories of personhood, self-identity and gender identity are produced and reproduced through engagement with the world.

Anthropologists have been very reluctant, until recently, to discuss either the development of self-identity or the development of gender identity. The reasons for this have clearly been both technical and theoretical, although anthropologists have frequently preferred to present the difficulty solely as a technical problem: 'we cannot get inside the heads of actors'. This representation of the problem as primarily a technical one is quite misleading. In fact, the overwhelming difficulty is one of under-theorisation, and could be directly addressed by the development both of a theory of the subject and of a theory of the acquisition of subjectivity. In so far as anthropologists have discussed the acquisition of subjectivity and gender identity, they have tended to base their work on a straightforward theory of socialisation. Socialisation has been seen to be effected largely through child-rearing practices or through ritual activities, such as initiation. Work in this area has frequently been very functionalist, especially in the past, where it tended to imply a situation in which society had need of particular sorts of acculturated persons, who were rather uncomplicatedly female or male. Gender identity was certainly thought to be culturally constructed, but it was conceived of, in the end, as little more than a self-evident outcome of sexual differentiation. The theoretical underpinnings of this work tended to be a rather crude Freudianism mixed with object-relations theory and some developmental psychology. Recent work in the discipline is much more sensitive to issues of gender identity, and much of it focuses on pre-Oedipal dynamics and the repudiation of initial maternal attachment by male children (see, for example, Herdt, 1982, 1984). However, there is, as yet, very little cross-cultural work on female children and pre-Oedipal dynamics.

PSYCHOANALYSIS, LANGUAGE AND SUBJECTIVITY

Psychoanalysis has provided the humanities and the social sciences with an influential set of theories about the acquisition of subjectivity and gender identity. These theories have been exceedingly controversial, but they have proved persuasive because of the way in which they stress that feminine and masculine identities are not natural or given in biology, but must be constructed and should be understood therefore as cultural achievements. There has been considerable debate among feminist scholars as to whether or not Freud's account of the production of sexuality should be seen as an attempt to theorise gender identity on the basis of fixed psycho-sexual structures which have a single cause (e.g., the Oedipus complex). One of the issues at stake here is whether or not Freud's theory endorses patri-archal forms of heterosexuality, in the context of a theory of fixed sexual difference which postulates masculinity as the norm (e.g., Mitchell, 1974; Mitchell and Rose, 1982; Rose, 1986).

More recently, a number of scholars have drawn on Lacan's re-reading of Freud and on various post-Lacanian theories. These theories are attrac-tive because they emphasise the crucial role which language plays in the construction of personal identity. Lacan's theory of the constitution of the subject in language explicitly questions dominant notions of the subject in philosophy, sociology and psychology. Lacan argues that the constitution of self is bound up with the world of images and representations and thus the self has no essential qualities, since it is not born, but made. A key point in the construction of the Lacanian subject is the mirror stage. This stage is an account of the primal separation of mother and child, and marks the child's entry into what Lacan calls the Imaginary order, as well as laying the foundations for social and linguistic identity. The mirror stage, which takes place between 6 and 18 months, begins with the child's recognition of its image in a mirror. The child identifies with the image and internalises it. The internalised image or imago provides the child with a sense of wholeness and completeness, and it introduces the child to an idea of its separateness from others. However, this sense of wholeness is illusory because it conflicts with the child's fragmented and fragmentary experi-ence of its body. This fragmentation is the result of the fact that different parts of the body mature at different rates. Furthermore, Lacan is at pains to emphasise that the self is always a split self, and it must logically be so because it is based on a relationship between ego and alter-ego. Lacan argues that the subject, to be a subject at all, must internalise otherness as a condition of its possibility. This is because it is by identifying and incor-porating the image of itself, which is also the image of another, that the child begins to represent itself to itself. The result of this is that, while the ego sees itself as its unified image, it is in fact split, internally divided between self and other (Grosz, 1990: 30–5).

In developing this account of the mirror stage, Lacan is emphasising that the ego is not self-contained and autonomous, but is intersubjective and depends on its relations with the other. He argues further that the ego is not dominated by reality, but rather by representation and modes of identification. The result is a subject which takes itself as its own object and which remains split. Thus Lacan disputes the assumption of a fixed, unified and naturally given identity at the core of the subject, while arguing that the subject's capacity to know itself and know the world is not dominated by reality, but by the ego's investment in certain images and representations (Grosz, 1990: 48).

Lacan's account of the mirror stage also raises interesting questions regarding the relationship between embodiment and identity. The notion that the formation of the ego is related to a recognition of the bodily image of another, which is also an image of itself, clearly means that the formation of the ego is directly linked to an image of the body's surface. It is by recognising this body-image that the subject distinguishes itself from its world. However, this body is not simply a physical body, but a 'lived anatomy' and one regulated by social, symbolic and cultural significations (Grosz, 1990: 43–4). It is a psychic map of the body, what Lacan calls the 'imaginary anatomy', and it varies with different cultural ideas about the body and biology. This body-image which is part of self identity is theorised by Lacan as neither mind nor body, neither natural nor cultural, but a threshold term, something which simultaneously occupies both positions (Grosz, 1990: 46).

It is quite clear that Lacan's theory of the subject and of the relationship between identity and embodiment seems potentially much more appropriate for understanding non-western views of the self, like those discussed above, than the conventional realist interpretations of Freud. However, the most valuable part of Lacan's theory for anthropologists is perhaps the part of his argument concerned with language, and with the importance of systems of meaning and signification for the constitution of subjectivity. Lacan's account of the child's entry into language involves the passage from the Imaginary order to the Symbolic. Lacan regards the mirror stage and the Imaginary order as sexually undifferentiated, and the child's acquisition of a sexual identity occurs only with its entry into the Symbolic. Entry into the Symbolic order is necessary for development and growth, because left alone the mother–child relation would provide an enclosed, circular relation which would make relations with a third, that is social relations, impossible (Grosz, 1990: 50). According to Lacan, a third term is necessary for social, linguistic and economic exchange to take place (Grosz, 1990: 67). This third term is the Symbolic father, representing the law prohibiting incest. The Oedipus complex is the point at which this third term intervenes in the mother–child dyad, and the child acquires a sexual identity, through the repudiation of the mother as love object and acquiescence to the law of the father. As a result of the Oedipalisation process, the child acquires a speaking position, a place in culture.

According to Lacan, the privileged signifier of the Symbolic order is the phallus, and sexual difference is constituted with reference to this key signifier. Thus, feminine and masculine positions, 'being' and 'having' the phallus, are not the product of biology, but of the system of significations, that is, of language. The phallus, as a signifier, is an element of language, which circulates within the system of significations, and should not be confused with the penis. However, Lacan's positioning of the phallus as the guarantor of meaning and as the crucial signifier which represents the distinction between the sexes has led to a heated debate about whether or not Lacan's theory is phallocentric (Gallop, 1982; Irigaray, 1985; Ragland-Sullivan, 1986; Mitchell and Rose, 1982). The charges of phallocentrism certainly seem justified on at least three counts. First, Lacan, like Freud, provides a much more convincing account of the acquisition of a sexed subject position for males than for females. Second, by Lacan's own admission, the recognition of different sexed subject positions, consequent on the threat of castration, is a consequence of the fact that each sex confuses the phallic signifier with a part or the whole of its body. In this process, the male and the female acquire a position, *vis-à-vis* the key signifier, as either having the phallus (for the male) or being the phallus (for the female). The male has the phallus because he has a penis, while the female is the phallus because she is castrated and becomes the object of man's desire, a phallus for him. The whole theory thus rests, in spite of protestations to the contrary, on considerable theoretical and psychic elision between the penis and the phallus. Third, Lacan provides no convincing account of why the phallus should be the key signifier of the Symbolic order, nor why it should stand as the mark of sexual difference.

The positive aspects of Lacan's work are that he has suggested a socio-linguistic theory of subjectivity, which enables female and male subjects to be seen as the product of social, historical and cultural systems of signification, rather than as biological entities. His theory of the symbolic emphasises that language, law and symbolic exchange are at the basis of society and social order. Finally, his emphasis on a subject defined by and in language reverses the causal relationship which social science habitually poses between subjectivity and language. Instead of a subject which speaks, and which is the source and author of meaning and discourse, Lacan proposes a subject which is articulated by language itself, and is the site of representations, inscriptions and meanings (Grosz, 1990: 148).

LACAN AND ANTHROPOLOGY

In terms of the application of Lacanian ideas to ethnographic data, there is as yet very little to go on. There are certainly a large number of societies which emphasise the importance of detaching male children from their mothers and from the world of women, which is also sometimes spoken of as pre-social in some sense. There are many instances in the ethnographic record of societies which associate identity and sociality with language and language use. However, to make anything of these generalities much more systematic work would need to be done.

Amelia Bell is one anthropologist who has investigated the links between subjectivity, gender and language among the Creek Indians of north-eastern Oklahoma. Her findings are very interesting. She notes that, for Creeks, language originates in a baby without form or shape and flows in babbles. In this state, language is referred to as female. When a child is born it is said to know everything because 'it is still connected to the female "watery funda-ment" before birth, in which universal knowledge exists'. Until the child talks, it is carried by women because 'it has no bones'. When it starts to speak coherently, it is said to have bones and must walk by itself (Bell, 1990: 338). The act of speaking forces an initial separation between child and mother. According to Bell, Creek babies of both sexes are said to be female because they lack bones, and, by metaphorical extension, the phallus. Through Creek myths which emphasise the role of a male definitional power in separating and defining a primordial, generative power which is female, and through ideas which associate social reproduction with the male ability to arrest and define the flow of uncontrolled female productivity, a notion of a male signifier which marks the transition from an undifferentiated to a differentiated state emerges. Self-identity and gender identity are associated with the acquisition of speech and with the entrance into a sociocultural and linguistic order which is defined by the phallus.

Bell elaborates on this point by making it clear that self-identity and gender identity are constructed in discourse, not only through local ideas about gender relations, social reproduction and the nature of people's relation to the world, but also through various practical activities. Such activities include gender-differentiated tasks whose successful perform-ance is thought to be connected to the essential nature of particular sorts of gendered persons. For example, the skill of good cooking is thought to inhere in a woman, and a woman who cannot cook is thought to have been afflicted by 'bad medicine' (Bell, 1990: 335). However, the most important activity is speech itself. Creek women and men have a different relation-ship to language and to language use. Women's speech is typified as flowing and uncontrolled, and women do not speak in most public and ritual contexts. Women apparently 'freely assent to withhold their speech in these public contexts as a sign that they are not dangerous', that their generative capacities are defined and under control (Bell, 1990: 338).

Considered in the light of Lacanian theories of the construction of the subject and of subjectivity, Bell's ethnography is suggestive. However, it cannot be said to prove or disprove Lacan's ideas. Lacan's theory and Bell's ethnography are probably best considered as parallel discourses on subjectivity and gender identity which give mutual insight into each other. Part of the difficulty in applying Lacanian ideas to ethnographic material concerns the question of what is meant by saying that the subject is constituted in language. Lacan is clear on this point and emphasises that when he says language he does not mean social discourse, he means instead a system of signification, a system of differences. Lacan is able to maintain this position because, although his theory is a theory of the social constitution of the subject, it is not a theory which takes account of social institutions, social practices, local power relations and social discourses. The Lacanian subject is an abstracted, if not actually an abstract, subject. This point connects to Lacan's concept of the subject itself. The subject should not be confused either with the person or with the self. The assumption of a sexed subject position is a prerequisite for agency and for self-identity, but it is not a description of the individual or self. Subjectivity is best understood as an attribute of the self. It is for this reason that Lacanian theory ultimately gives us very little insight into the experience of being a gendered individual. To understand that experience, it is necessary to link Lacanian ideas about the constitution of subjectivity to social discourses and discursive practices. This involves linking the assumption of a sexed subject position to all the potential sexed subject positions which are available in social life and social practice. It matters, therefore, that people have local views of the person, of the sort of people women and men are meant to be, of the nature of the biological make-up of the physical being, of the relations between the human and non-human worlds and many other local theories, and are able to use these ideas to reflect on the nature of their experience and on the kind of person/self they believe themselves to be. The assumption of a sexed subject position makes sense only in the context of social discourses and discursive practices; without this context there would be no potential or necessity for any sort of subject, precarious or otherwise.

Recent feminist theory has sought to make use of Lacanian ideas in precisely this way, and to utilise the concept of the non-essentialist subject constituted in language to try to come to grips with individuals' experiences of being gendered subjects. The important point here is to examine how we are all subject to discourse and to the various subject positions which are made available to us in discourse. Such subject positions can be resisted, both consciously and unconsciously, but it is in relation to these positions, even if in contradiction with them, that we construct a sense of ourselves as selves, as individuals and as persons.

However, once we begin to consider the constitution of the subject within social discourses and discursive practices, the social, historical and cultural contingency of subjectivity is brought to the fore. Psychoanalytic theory, including Lacanian theory, postulates a narrative of the acquisition of sexuality and subjectivity which rests on the presumption of a fixed psycho-sexual order. In other words, Lacan proposes universal structures and processes within which individuals acquire a precarious sexuality and subjectivity, one which is constantly threatened by the return of the repressed. However, this gendered subjectivity is none the less brought about by a fixed set of structures and processes, and all existing social relations must themselves be read in terms of those structures and processes (Weedon, 1987: 56). For anthropologists, there is no reason why the law of the father, to which Lacan refers, should be universal. In fact, it seems more sensible to assume that this law is open to cultural reformulation. This is most evident when we turn to look at alternative conceptions of gender and gender identity. Lacan, like Freud, assumes that the assumption of a sexed subject position is possible only in terms of a fixed binarism – to 'be' or to 'have' the phallus. There is no reason, as discussed earlier, why the phallus should everywhere and always be the key signifier of sexual difference, but nor is there any reason to suppose that sexual difference should always and everywhere be constructed in terms of a binary relation between two mutually exclusive categories. If we assume that local discourses on gender and gender identity make a difference to the way people think of gender and gender identity, then we cannot afford to assume that binary exclusivity modelled on external genitalia necessarily provides an appropriate model for understanding sexual difference and gender identity around the world.

What Lacanian theory offers social anthropology is a theory of the subject and of the acquisition of gendered subjectivity. It moves anthropological theory away from a reliance on essentialist and fixed views of the nature of the person and the self, and brings out the enormous potential which exists in cross-cultural data for reflection on these issues. Social anthropology in its turn provides a critique of psychoanalytic theory, and of the assumption of universalistic psycho-sexual structures, and emphasises instead the importance of constructing a theory of the subject and of subjectivity which takes into account the social discourses and discursive practices which provide the context in which we all ultimately become gendered subjects.

NOTES

1 The only notable exceptions in this regard are recent studies in that area of ethnopsychology which has become known as the anthropology of emotion; see Abu-lughod, 1986; Lutz, 1988.
2 A great deal of new research from Melanesia does deal with problems of identity and sexual difference for males. See Herdt, 1982, 1984; Herdt and Stoler, 1990.
3 McHugh has recently made this point using data on the Gurungs of Nepal and contra Dumont and Marriott (McHugh, 1989). Gewertz has also recently criticised Margaret Mead and Nancy Chodorow, who uses Mead's original data, for assessing the strength and weaknesses of Tchambuli women in terms of their ability to individuate or act as individuals. Gewertz's argument is simply that such an approach is ethnocentric (Gewertz, 1984).
4 I am greatly indebted to Judith Butler. Her work on gender identity has provided the inspiration for my argument in this section (Butler, 1990).

COMMENT

Florence Bégoin-Guignard

Although the subject of psychoanalysis is sexuality, not all the implications which follow from the differences between the sexes are recognised in the original Freudian parameters. Despite post-Freudian contributions, especially those of Klein and other women analysts, the implicit model which still prevails today in the 'society' – in the ethnographic sense of the word – of psychoanalysts is that of a *small Oedipal boy of 3 to 4 years old*. The Lacanian movement, which has had its hour of glory in France, has only served to make this model more rigid, taking no account of the truly deep changes in social organisation which have occurred since Freud.

Thus there is much to say on the latent significance of the sacrosanct 'law of the father', which is supposed to separate the mother from the child and therefore, from the manifest point of view, prohibits heterosexual incest for the boy and homosexual incest for the girl. To take this law literally is to forget that the infantile desire of the father is also realised in it, in the return of the repressed from his own childhood: 'You took my mother away from me, I take her back from you' – implying thus a conflation of mother/wife. So one might oppose the mythical Oedipus with 'his swollen feet' to an Oedipus with 'little feet', an adult man who uses the power bestowed upon him by the law which he himself has established, in order to evade it by giving his transgression the appearance of legitimacy.

In dealing with the person, this paper not only raises the question of individuation but equally the questions of splitting and identifications, and particularly the balance between different types of identifications. On the issue of physical embodiment, I would suggest that, from a psychoanalytic point of view, the *cogito ergo sum* cannot constitute a model for physical and sexual embodiment because, even in the west, sexual identity is far from being a stable attribute of an individual. Without considering the subject of transsexuality there is no need to evoke either a psychotic or a classic neurotic patient to find an important, though subtle, problematic concerning sexual identity in every human being.

Admittedly, there are many 'muddles in the model' within psychoanalytic thought, which is an evolving model which resists change at many points. So, even while the Lacanian additions are interesting, they are far from providing a complete solution. In particular, Lacan makes an error in considering the self as a whole, not split; the only split considered being that which separates the self from the non-self, forgetting in this way the Freudian advance on the splitting of the ego.

In this respect, the Lacanian theory of 'incompleteness of being', even if it is correct as a metaphor for a desire, contributes to disguising the problem of identity, whether it be of sex or gender. Accepting that 'object relation' and 'identification' are two sides of one and the same process of humanisation, the real problematic is that of the nature, quality and complexity of a) the splitting which results in the primary psychic formations of 'being in the world' and b) the identifications which attach themselves to these primary formations.

Based on the first Freudian elaborations concerning the process of 'mentalisation', knowing the system of 'representation of things – representation of words', the Lacanian theorisation of the imaginary and the symbolic, and of the necessity of language in order to pass from one to the other, may appear as an acceptable paraphrase from the Freudian point of view if one is considering the primary relationship which exists for the human being between language and thought. However, this theory reveals itself as completely erroneous in view of the laws which rule psychic development when, by reducing the mother to an imaginary category, it therefore denies her all psychic life and, particularly, all the post-Oedipal organisation of the adult. Such an organisation inevitably implies: firstly, introjective identifications of the mother to her own father and to his penis; secondly, projective identifications to her mate, who in the best case is the father of her child; thirdly, projective identifications to her sexed child. Thus, it is from her situation as an adult woman, post-Oedipal and sexual, that the mother is engaged with her child and speaks to him or her.

It would be a pity if anthropologists were to follow Lacan in the confusion he makes at this point between the Oedipal triangle and the social group. In the light of this distinction, I would agree with Moore who considers that those societies which impose a premature separation of the small boy from his mother can be classified as pre-social. I think that they are equally pre-Oedipal, because here the symbolisation of the link between mother and son is absent and aborted. The obvious hypothesis that this relates to the denial by the group of the existence of any psychic life for women should not lead us, however, to confound Oedipal and group processes.

In conclusion, the apparent simplicity of the concept of gender identity in the west seems to me to be an illusion coming from the greater complexity and the lesser ritualisation of the social expressions of gender ambiguity. French works (for example, David, 1971) on bisexuality show clearly that the problem has been considered. From my point of view, any too rigid state of equilibrium between the feeling of belonging to one biological sex and identifications towards the opposite sex constitute for an individual a psychopathologic risk.

BIBLIOGRAPHY

Abu-Lughod, L. (1986) *Veiled Sentiments: Honor and Poetry in a Bedouin Society.* Berkeley: University of California Press.
Atkinson, J. (1990) 'How gender makes a difference in Wana society', in J. Atkinson and S. Errington (eds) *Power and Difference: Gender in Island Southeast Asia.* Stanford, CA: Stanford University Press.
Bell, A. R. (1990) 'Separate people: speaking of Creek men and women', *American Anthropologist* 92: 332–45.
Bourdieu, P. (1976) *Outline of a Theory of Practice.* Cambridge: Cambridge University Press.
—— (1990) *The Logic of Practice.* Cambridge: Polity Press.
Butler, J. (1990) *Gender Trouble: Feminism and the Subversion of Identity.* London: Routledge.
David, C. (1971) *La bisexualité psychique.* Paris: PUF.
Dieterlen, G. (1941) *Les Ames des Dogon.* Paris: Institut d'Ethnologie (Travaux et memoires, 40).
Dumont, L. (1970) *Homo Hierarchicus: The Caste System and its Implications.* London: Weidenfeld & Nicolson.
Flax, J. (1987) 'Postmodernism and gender relations in feminist theory', *Signs* 12(4): 621–43.
Fortes, M. (1973) 'On the concept of the person among the Tallensi', in G. Dieterlen (ed.) *Colloque International sur le Notion de Personne en Afrique.* Paris: CRNS.
Gallop, J. (1982) *Feminism and Psychoanalysis: The Daughter's Seduction.* London: Macmillan.
Gewertz, D. (1984) 'The Tchambuli view of persons: a critique of individualism in the works of Mead and Chodorow', *American Anthropologist* 86: 615–29.
Grosz, E. (1990) *Jacques Lacan: A Feminist Introduction.* London: Routledge.
Hallowell, A. I. (1971) *Culture and Experience.* New York: Schocken.
Heelas, P. and Lock, A. (eds) (1981) *Indigenous Psychologies: The Anthropology of the Self.* London: Academic Press.
Herdt, G. (ed.) (1982) *Rituals of Manhood: Male Initiation in New Guinea.* Berkeley: University of California Press.

—— (1984) *Ritualised Homosexuality in Melanesia*. Berkeley: University of California Press.

Herdt, G. and Stoller, R. (1990) *Intimate Communications: Erotics and the Study of Culture*. New York: Columbia University Press.

Irigaray, L. (1985) *This Sex Which Is Not One*. Ithaca: Cornell University Press.

Lacan, J. (1977) *Ecrits: A Selection*. London: Tavistock.

Leenhardt, M. (1979) [1947] *Do Kamo: Person and Myth in the Melanesian World*. Chicago: University of Chicago Press.

Lévi-Strauss, C. (1969) *The Elementary Structures of Kinship*. Boston: Beacon Press.

Lienhardt, G. (1985) 'Self: public, private. Some African representations', in M. Carrithers *et al.* (eds) *The Category of the Person*. Cambridge: Cambridge University Press.

Lutz, C. (1988) *Unnatural Emotions: Everyday Sentiments on a Micronesian Atoll and their Challenge to Western Theory*. Chicago: University of Chicago Press.

McHugh, E. (1989) 'Concepts of the person among the Gurungs of Nepal', *American Ethnologist* 16(1): 75–86.

Marriott, K. (1976) 'Hindu transactions: diversity without duration', in B. Kapferer (ed.) *Transactions and Meanings*. Philadelphia: Institute for the Study of Human Values.

Mead, G. H. (1934) *Mind, Self and Society*. Chicago: University of Chicago Press.

Meigs, A. (1990) 'Multiple gender ideologies and statuses', in P. Sanday (ed.) *Beyond the Second Sex: New Directions in the Anthropology of Gender*. Philadelphia: University of Pennsylvania Press.

Mitchell, J. (1974) *Psychoanalysis and Feminism*. Harmondsworth: Penguin.

Mitchell, J. and Rose, J. (1982) *Feminine Sexuality: Jacques Lacan and the Ecole Freudienne*. London: Macmillan.

Ragland-Sullivan, E. (1986) *Jacques Lacan and the Philosophy of Psychoanalysis*. Urbana: University of Illinois Press.

Rose, J. (1986) *Sexuality in the Field of Vision*. London: Verso.

Smith, J. (1981) 'Self and experience in Maori culture', in P. Heelas and A. Lock (eds) *The Anthropology of the Self*. London: Academic Press.

Strathern, M. (1988) *The Gender of the Gift*. Berkeley: University of California Press.

Strauss, A. (1982) 'The structure of the self in Northern Cheyenne culture', in B. Lee (ed.) *Psychosocial Theories of the Self*. New York: Plenum Press.

Tress, D. M. (1988) 'Comment on Glax's "Postmodernism and gender relations in feminist theory",' *Signs* 14(1): 196–203.

Weedon, C. (1987) *Feminist Practice and Poststructuralist Theory*. Oxford: Blackwell.

Whitehead, H. (1981) 'The bow and the burdenstrap: a new look at institutionalised homosexuality in native North America', in S. Ortner and H. Whitehead (eds) *Sexual Meanings: The Cultural Construction of Gender and Sexuality*. Cambridge: Cambridge University Press.

Yanagisako, S. and Collier, J. (1987) 'Toward a unified analysis of gender and kinship', in J. Collier and S. Yanagisako (eds) *Gender and Kinship: Essays Toward a Unified Analysis*. Stanford, CA: Stanford University Press.

9　Lacanian ethnopsychoanalysis

Charles-Henry Pradelles de Latour

Lacan shifted the focus of Freudian psychoanalytic theory by concentrating on the issue of the subject. He stands apart from his contemporaries in draining the latter notion of its normal meanings. From his standpoint, the subject is no longer the philosopher's perception-cum-consciousness, nor the moralist's intentionality, nor again the hidden being of depth psychology. It is rather linked to an original lack, an absence of being and substance which lies at the very origin of desire, in so far as this is distinguishable from need or demand. Whereas need is governed by the interplay of satisfaction and the lack thereof, and demand (which essentially is a demand for love) suspends such interplay in order to relocate it in some unattainable though compulsively yearned-for hereafter, desire itself is never brought to a close by any satisfaction or failure to satisfy. Desire, by which Lacan means to desire something other than the object required to satisfy a need, finds its completion in that which is not actively wanted. Where there is a lack, there is also a desire and a subject. In other words, the subject's failure is to be superfluously present, being more than it is, and looking for guarantees when at bottom there are none to offer.

　　Subject and desire thus do not correspond to any kind of simple opposition such as truth and falsehood, or any other such binary mental schema, but rather to a ternary grouping as with the ego, id and super-ego introduced by Freud in his second topos, and taken up by Lacan in his three 'dimensions': the imaginary, the real and the symbolic. Such a treatment sees the subject as deriving from a third party termed the capital-Other, the Other of language, hence the 'I' who both speaks and listens. This entirely conjectural Other is essentially a symbolic locus which 'ex-ists' (i.e., is posited as external to the subject) both by its presence and its absence. Since it cannot be defined in terms of being or not-being, it cannot be mistaken for God or used to underwrite any idea. It can no more authenticate good faith than it can bad faith.

　　Discussing Lacanian ethnopsychoanalysis, therefore, means considering an ethnology that tackles the problem of the subject and the Other. Such an approach involves not simply ordering the material data according to binary schemata – cause and effect, means and end – nor using sets or simple classificatory oppositions, such as the individual and society, nature and culture, *langue* and *parole*. It must also involve bringing out the ternary features of the data. We shall here outline the early stages in this process by examining how the subject is established from the three Oedipal phases. To bring out more clearly the way in which the ternary nature of the subject contrasts with the duality of the self, we shall first consider the 'mirror phase' in the formation of the self. The interlocking of the subject and society at every stage will be stressed by showing that in the matrilineal kinship system of the Trobrianders, familiar to anthropologists, every stage in the development of a subject is closely associated with clearly defined sociological facts.

THE MIRROR PHASE

The main characteristic of the newborn child's bodily being is its total detachment from all the surrounding world except its mother. This disjunction between the *Innenwelt* and the *Umwelt* is revealed during the early neonatal months in the signs of discomfort and the inchoate gestures which are attributable to a lack of motor co-ordination (Lacan, 1966). Around the fifth or sixth month, when the child can first recognise its image in a mirror held up to it, the captured reflection is greeted with a bright-eyed gaze and radiant mimicry: confirmation that it is beginning to conceive of itself as a unified whole, thanks to this first identification, which thus marks a victory over the previously dismembered state of the body. This imago, in the fullest sense of that word, is a genuine idol or Gestalt matrix, through which the self conceives of itself as a unity and prefigures, as though in a mirage, its maturing powers and the coming co-ordination of its limbs. In the last analysis, however, the imago, which is the origin of the self, comes from a mere fiction, from a mirror-game played with the child by those around it. Thus the self is not formed, as Freud thought, by moving from the inward towards an outward projection of the self, but by moving in the opposite direction, with the external and social seen as primary and the very foundation of inwardness.

There is, then, in Lacan's view, no primordial auto-erotism, since it is on the other-self, or the imago, that primary process and narcissistic tensions are both grounded. 'The other by its image simultaneously attracts and repels me; I am only through the other and yet at the same time it remains *alienus*, foreign; this other which is myself and other than myself' (Julien, 1985: 50). The fascinations of love and the tensions of jealousy are already at work therein, for the imago, in constantly switching between the two alternative poles (if not self then the other), already lies at the base of the future reciprocity between the self and others.

Though richly suggestive, this Gestalt remains incomplete, which is why Lacan (1966) compares it to a crutch or a prosthetic limb, that first straightens the body, then takes its weight and helps it to adopt to an upright posture and learn to walk. The imago is not a piece of passive reflection but a morphogenetic act, enabling a bodily development based upon an erectile form and upright stature, most perfectly exemplified by the ambivalent fate of Lot's wife, simultaneously turned to stone and eternalised, at once dead and immortal. This phallic form, with which to varying degrees we all (men and women) identify, is universal, and can be found, as Malinowski (1922, 1935) claims, around the world in standing stones, towers, masts, magic wands and pointed bones. For this same reason it also becomes the main support for the stiffly erected ideal-self, which is why everyone sees themselves not only as other, but as superior to others.

This ideal-self – directly linked with the imago – which lies at the heart of resemblance and in which we recognise ourselves, thus becomes for us the threshold of the visible world, beyond which lie in shadow those comic or tragic apparitions – look-alikes, automata, *doppelgangers* – which emphasise the otherness of the self. The doubles who inhabit the realms of the dead and scenes of witchcraft are all the more disturbing in that they recall the unbearable strangeness of the ego to itself. In the Trobriands, the dead separate into different aspects, as both mischievous ghosts known as *kosi* which haunt the home for a period after a death and as enduring spirits, the *baloma*, which appear in dreams (Malinowski, 1948), while witches turn into fireflies, nightjars, or else clone themselves into high-speed beings who sit astride ropes and fly through the air (Malinowski, 1922).

This imaginary mirror-image which is the main component of the self is a keystone of numerous beliefs and kinship systems. Trobrianders claim that they look like their fathers, with whom they share no blood, and not like their maternal uncles, with whom they do. From this, we see that the child identifies with the father, both physically and personally, in a more formative way than with the uncle. Thus, it can be observed with Powell (1956: 134) that the father is not as foreign to his children as Malinowski (1932) asserts.

THE MOTHER OBJECT AND FRUSTRATION

The relationship of the newborn child with those around it is governed not only by the forming of the imago, but also and simultaneously by its bodily relation to a privileged object upon which nutritional life depends: the breast and its substitutes. When the child is hungry it cries, when its hunger is satisfied it falls asleep. This need-driven behaviour soon becomes more complex, with the real object being linked to the affective presence of the mother. When the breast in this way becomes a token of trust, a sign of love granted or withheld, the child tends to vary its mirror activities in order to control the comings and goings of its mother; to the infant she becomes the first symbol (present/absent) that it can make its own. If the mother does not succumb to its advances, she lapses in the child's esteem, but she thereby also proves herself to be a real power, all the more powerful in that the infant's nutritional and affective life is dependent upon her whims (Lacan, 1958).

From this point onwards, needing and wanting love are tightly inter-locked, with the result that the frustrations of love can be compensated for by the satisfaction of needs (as in bulimia, for example) and the frustration of needs (anorexia being only one such case) can be used to heighten the value of the love at stake (Lacan, 1956–7). It is in this way that the immediate object of a drive is subordinated to the search for an ambivalent, simultaneously enchanted and tyrannical, symbolic object – to be found somewhere beyond the mother, within the realm of the Other, in the form of infallible magic objects or omnipotent mythical beings. It is because subject and object are not yet separated that this space is inhabited by animal totems and fairies, ogres and monsters, and the multifarious mis-shapen creatures that all oral literatures evoke.

The infant's primary relationship with its mother has sociological impli-cations that are well exemplified in the Trobriands by the affective and bodily links uniting members of the same matrilineage. Membership of the same uterine family is reinforced by magical formulas, land-ownership and obligations of solidarity, as in any corporate group. It is also expressed in some exceptionally powerful metaphors: 'to be of the same flesh and blood', 'to make one body' (Malinowski, 1932), or even 'to suckle the same breast' (Weiner, 1976). The counterparts of these are death and bodily decomposition: one cannot touch the corpse of a blood relative without the risk of a serious illness or an early end (Malinowksi, 1932). This blood bond that knows no death is based on a common line of ascent through which members of the same matrilineage are all related to one ancestral couple, a woman and her brother(s) who, according to legend, emerged from a cave with all the magic needed to cultivate land and live in society (Malinowski, 1926). Members of the same matrilineage therefore are related beyond their mothers to mythical figures believed to be omni-potent and eternal. These ancestors, known as *tosonapulo*, are remembered by their personal names, which are often incanted at the beginning of magical spells. They are supposed to have the maternal symbolic object *par excellence*.

NAMES-OF-THE-FATHER AND DEPRIVATION

For Freud the central phase of the Oedipus complex occurs when the infant turns away from its mother to identify with its father. Although this identification with an idealised male figure is laden with potential hostility, it serves to detach the child from its mother and, in so doing, institutes the incest taboo (Freud, 1923). Lacan develops this theory by emphasising the mother's role and by insisting on the symbolic nature of the identification with the father. If the infant were to remain the sole object of all the mother's desires, it might well remain bound in an exclusive dual relationship, dominated by capricious and omnipotent figures. To avoid this danger, with its potential for madness, the mother must accordingly desire something other than the infant; thus, the privileged object of her desire is situated away from herself, and towards the father. However, this veiled and inaccessible paternal object (known as the phallus) towards which the infant's desire is drawn can be apprehended only via the mediating devices that Lacan terms Names-of-the-Father. The capital N and the hyphens show that these names are the equivalent of proper names, though they are not necessarily homophonically identical to any family patronymics. For every subject the Names-of-the-Father are different and, although there may be two or three of them, sometimes overlapping, one of them will tend to dominate the others, hence the use of the term in the singular in normal usage. Like all proper names, the Name-of-the-Father cannot be translated and it conveys more a reference than a meaning. What it does denote, however, is not so much the person of the father as the object of the mother's desire, but rather the referent which unconsciously endows the father with value for the mother.

The Name-of-the-Father thus lets the infant make the transition from autonomous demand to heteronomous desire; from a dual relationship centred on the mother object (the breast) to a tripartite relation focused around an object referring to the father. Replacing an internal maternal object by an external paternal one is both an act of deprivation and a displacement. It deprives the capital-Other of the phallus, the original symbolic object on which the mother's omnipotence relied, and it relocates the privileged object of desire in the id, a both real and imaginary beyond, which is external to the locus of the Other, the place of language (see diagram L below). By being detached from the original symbolic object, the capital-Other is instantly deprived of all power, becoming no more than a torn locus, known as the barred-Other, through which the child can enter only as the subject of desire. What the subject and desire have in common is this separation between two orders: the Other and the objects of drives stemming from the id. In relation to the symbolic Other, both subject and desire derive from a lack that ensures their multiple meanings and constant renewal; as part of the reality external to the language, they are secretly activated by incomplete and uncontrollable drives from the id. Unlike the self, the subject of desire is not a unity or condensation of meaning but rather a split and a loss of meaning.

In a similar way the total group of subjects, which Lacan calls the 'collectivity' (which is different from the collective unconscious), relies on a lack of relationship that is the very basis of separation and otherness. In the Trobriands this collectivity is unambiguously made up of the father's relatives and relatives by marriage. If blood relatives are focused around ingestible nourishment, such as yams, whose richness is matrilineally internal (auto-reproducible), father's relatives, on the other hand, are privileged by the association with ornaments and external wealth, such as shells, which favour seduction and sexual relationships. Moreover, whereas blood relatives may not approach their dead, father's relatives and other relatives by marriage have the dreaded task of conducting all the funeral rites in order to detach the dead from their matrilineage so that they may become *baloma*, or mortal ancestors (Weiner, 1987). In such a society, therefore, blood relatives (maternal uncles) are unifiers, while relatives by marriage (fathers) are separators.

The symbolic intermediaries with whom children identify in order to detach themselves from their mother thus refer not to the maternal uncle but to the father who, as relative by marriage, is external to the mother's matrilineage. Thus the Name-of-the-Father both deprives and displaces, as with westerners, except that in this case it is not the matrilineage of the mother which loses its origins, but that of the father, whose biological paternity is unacknowledged. Much has been written on this belief (especially, Leach, 1967; Spiro, 1968, 1982), but in this particular social context it implies that agnatic descendants of the father's matrilineage cannot inherit the maternal object, represented both by the maternal flesh and by the child's spirit, *waiwaia*, which are transmitted through the uterine line. In other words, there is no link between the father's ancestors and his children. If, then, the Other that is the mother and the maternal uncle is centred around the *tosonapulo*, or omnipotent founding ancestors, the barred-Other, who is unconnected to any origins and bereft of power, is represented by the *baloma* of the father, the mortal forefathers who have no magical powers (Malinowski, 1948). It is when confronted by this external third party that children enter as subjects, and join the collectivity which is deprived of origin. This absence of origin which here differentiates the father's and mother's matrilineages is equivalent to the incest taboo.

THE IDEAL-EGO AND CASTRATION

Delicate and ephemeral though it is, like any other symbol, the Name-of-the-Father is still the major signifier, 'the Name placed above every name that religion taught us to call upon. If it is not God, then it is god in every species or god in all his names' (Dufour, 1990: 312). In other words, it is a name that is trusted and that the subject depends upon in order to be able to trust others and to entertain reciprocal relationships. The Name-of-the-Father is, in this sense, the support to which the ideal-ego is anchored in one way or another; it is the singular signifier upon which any identification with others depends. The self-ideal, or bodily imago, in early acts of identification will henceforth be subordinated to the Other-level function of the ideal-ego in the symbolic order. It is thus that, as Lacan (1971) says, loving someone often means, in the final analysis, loving a name.

When the ideal-ego is under too much pressure, the imago of the self-ideal, which brought that idealisation into play, is put gravely to the test. To salvage the situation the super-ego has the task of censoring and sacrificing: a pathology which might result in symbolic or even actual amputation. To escape from this happening, the subject may resort to the symbolic destruction of idealisation. We know that in the course of an analysis we get to castration by replaying, through transference, the totality of our identifications, and by using words, particularly puns, to dismantle the creations of the unconsciousness. The Name-of-the-Father, which initially overwhelmed the alienated object of demand by being too strong, is then gradually de-idealised. The more it is relativised in comparison with other names, the more easily it can be placed within a series which is more open and livable. When the Name-of-the-Father is thus symbolically dead, being no longer alienably present, for any name that can be replaced may also be missing, then castration finally rejoins privation, in the absence of an original object.

In the Trobriands, as Melford Spiro (1982) has remarked, the ideal of the father lies at the base of that ambivalence between attraction and hostility which underlies father–son relationships. Since this ideal is not so strong as the maternal uncle ideal which is not deprived of origin, it helps those aspiring to climb the social hierarchy and become heads of their matri-lineage, village and finally cluster of villages (Powell, 1960). This ascent will involve difficulties and a certain narcissistic wounding. Only subjects firmly anchored in the resilient structure of desire can reach these positions and, by using exchange mechanism, stay at the head of a large clientele.

DIAGRAM L

Lacan plotted the four key points around which the self and the subject unfold on a graph known as diagram L (1966: 53, 571).

The binary-type self/other mirror relationship is shown by the upper diagonal axis, while the ternary nature of the subject is indicated, in two parts, by the diagonal axis passing beneath the former. Along the broken line the subject is split between the capital-Other (the symbolic order) and the id where the phallus, the object of the mother's desire (both real and imaginary), cannot be reached. The overlapping of the two diagonals, one passing under the other, reminds us that the subject belongs to a different location from the one in which everyday mirror relationships take place.

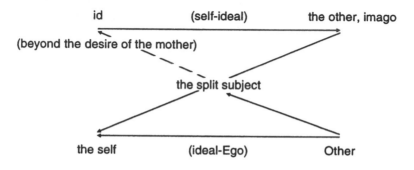

Diagram L

The upper and lower horizontal axes bring out similarities and differences, in parallels, between the self-ideal (upper side) focused on the other, and the ideal-ego (lower side) grafted on to the capital-Other. The self is rather like the subject normally split between these two ideals and is organised by them.

CONCLUSION

In Lacan's theory, the subject is thus a crucial yet open-ended problematic. So long as the subject remains unresolved, we can avoid substantifying the unconscious or trying to bring it back into the ground of the controllable, relating to some binary mental schema, such as the archaism and finality suggested in Ricoeur's (1965) hermeneutics, or the idiosyncratic ethnic personalities proposed by Devereux's (1951) ethnopsychiatry. According to Lacan, the unconscious is not grounded in some kind of primordial or ultimate meaning but, on the contrary, is constituted in an absence of meaning from which we emerge as a universal subject, for all the unique subjects who share the same lack are to that extent equal. This lack is linked

to the incest taboo and lies at the very foundations of sexuality – heteronomous desire – and the symbolic separation of the generations through
death. The collectivity or grouping of subjects from which sexual and
generational differences derive is therefore something without which no
society could survive or perpetuate itself. If, then, anthropology broadly
stresses that societies are determined by ideas, economic relationships and
parental interdependences, the task of ethnopsychoanalysis is to show that,
within these constraints, societies are based in the final analysis on an
absence, which indeed destroys any inter-subjectivity, each culture
handling this in its own way.

BIBLIOGRAPHY

Devereux, G. (1951) *Reality and Dream: The Psychotherapy of a Plains Indian*,
New York: International Universities Press.
Dufour, R. (1990) *Les Mystères de la trinité*. Paris: Gallimard.
Freud, S. (1923) 'La Disparition du complexe d'Oedipe', in *La Vie sexuelle*. Paris:
Seuil, 8th edn, 1989, pp. 117–23.
Julien, Ph. (1985) *Le Retour à Freud de Jacques Lacan. L'application au miroir*.
Toulouse: Eres.
Lacan, J. (1956–57) *La Relation d'objet*. Séminaire inédit.
—— (1957–58) *Les Formations de l'inconscient*. Séminaire inédit.
—— (1959–60) *L'Identification*. Séminaire inédit.
—— (1966) *Les Ecrits*. Paris: Seuil.
—— (1970–71) *D'un Discours qui ne serait pas du semblant*. Séminaire inédit.
—— (1974–75) *RSI (Réel, symbolique, imaginaire)*. Séminaire inédit.
Leach, E. R. (1967) 'Virgin birth', *Proceedings of the Royal Anthropological
Institute*: 39–49.
Malinowski, B. (1922) *Argonauts of the Western Pacific*. London: Routledge &
Kegan Paul.
—— (1926) *Crime and Custom in Savage Society*. London: Allen & Unwin.
—— (1932) *The Sexual Life of Savages in Northwestern Melanesia*. London:
Routledge & Kegan Paul.
—— (1935) *Coral Gardens and their Magic: A Study of the Methods of Tilling the
Soil and of Agricultural Rites in the Trobriand Islands*, Vol. I. London: Allen &
Unwin.
—— (1948) 'Baloma: the spirits of the dead in the Trobriand Islands', in *Magic,
Science and Religion and Other Essays*. Glencoe, Ill.: The Free Press.
Powell, H. A. (1956) 'An analysis of present day social structure in the Trobriand
Islands', unpublished Ph.D. dissertation, University of London.
—— (1960) 'Competitive leadership in Trobriand political organization', *Journal
of the Royal Anthropological Institute* 90: 118–45.
Ricoeur, P. (1965) *De l'interprétation. Essai sur Freud*. Paris: Seuil. Translated
into English as *Freud and Philosophy: An Essay on Interpretation*. New Haven:
Yale University Press, 1970.
Spiro, M. E. (1968) 'Virgin birth, parthenogenesis, and the physiological paternity:
an essay in cultural interpretation', *Man, n.s.* 3: 242–61.
—— (1982) *Oedipus in the Trobriands*, Chicago: University of Chicago Press.

162   *The Lacanian perspective*

Weiner, A. B. (1976) *Women of Value, Men of Renown: New Perspective in Trobriand Exchange*. Austin: University of Texas Press.
—— (1987) *The Trobrianders of Papua New Guinea*. New York and London: Holt, Rinehart & Winston.

10 Lacan and anthropology

Comments on Chapters 8 and 9

Bernard Doray

What would an anthropology that took seriously the theoretical perspectives of a Lacanian psychoanalysis be like? Let me begin with the
reductions in anthropological thought which Pradelles de Latour sees as a
result of the tendency to adopt binary oppositions (individual/society,
cause/effect, etc.). Pradelles reminds us that in the Lacanian perspective
there is a ternary structure to the subject as opposed to a 'duality of the
self'. This is important even though the abstractness of the formulation
makes it difficult to explain. Pradelles takes firstly the mirror stage which
produces an imago and a fiction and which Lacan has described as being at
the very threshold of the imaginary. For the child, the speculative game is
the point of entry into an active understanding of the world. And it is by the
effect of a movement which, Pradelles emphasises, does not result from an
interior psychological projection towards the exterior environment but
rather from an inverse movement which takes the external to be prior and
to be the foundation of the internal. Infantile 'narcissism', including all
primary processes within it, cannot therefore be considered a consequence
of the self-centredness which a small subject, clinging steadfastly to his
own autonomy, can oppose to the force of society. On the contrary, it is first
produced by a massive intrusion of the other-self into the very interior of
his own being.

The ascending line of human subjectivity is not only what Lacan
referred to ironically at some point as 'the sociological poem of self
autonomy', woven around the pioneer-like metaphor of the conquest and
expansion of frontiers. Rather, it is through a complex movement, whose
outcome is not obvious at the start, that the subject 'becomes', as it rids
itself of the archaic forms that held it, through a continuous process of
metamorphosis and recurrence which starts as the child enters the mirror
stage. In this complex process, the failure of the dualist illusion plays an
essential part. It is on renouncing the notion of sharing one body with the
archaic mother and on realising that the mutual possession on which the

dualist illusion is based is not unlimited, that the enchanted world where the self and the other were originally joined is shattered.

To move to the question of the phallus and to the feminist critique of the Lacanian theory discussed by Henrietta Moore. To summarise, the phallo-centricism of Lacan comes from the ambiguous position that Lacan assigns to the phallus. On the one hand, the phallus does not concern only men, and Pradelles reminds us that for Lacan the primordial imago in the mirror stage has an erect(ile) form, the support of the self-ideal or the 'statue self', for women-to-be as much as for men-to-be. It is 'the phallic form, with which to varying degrees we all identify'. On the other hand, the argument runs that Lacan accepted as natural the elision between the phallus and the penis, through which men claim to their own profit all collective wisdom.

In so doing, Lacan would cede a realism to a quasi-universal sexism and help, theoretically, to tip the balance of the symbolic clues in the social order on the side of masculinity. Frankly, to me, this critique seems to result from a narrow interpretation of Lacan. In Lacan's understanding, the transition from the register of being (to be the phallus, all-powerful, the self-ideal, etc.) to the register of having (to have a limited desire, rule-bound and sayable) is the very process through which the subject comes into being. It is therefore not without an important counter-sense that one can, from this, conceive of a mechanical distribution of individuals which casts as outside subjectivity one half of humanity: either having the phallus (for the male) or being the phallus (for the female). What, on the contrary, is an indispensable feature in the theoretical plan of Lacan is the fact that there is some asymmetry in the way in which the desire of men and the desire of women towards the phallus is articulated.

It is precisely because the 'phallus' is a masculine attribute that encountering its mystery breaks open the mother–child dyad, giving access to the symbolic world and liberating the child. In other words, in answer to the charge of phallocentrism (whatever is the phallus, central to the ideologies of masculine domination, doing in the middle of this theory?), I would argue that what is at stake when one talks of the phallus in the Lacanian context is immediately connected neither to the economy of symbolic attributions between the sexes nor to the social contradictions which result from gender inequality. By putting the principal accent on the function of the symbolic agency (the agency of the letter) in the structuring of the subjective, he firstly emphasises a contradiction which has nothing to do with sexual identity. It concerns the passage from the closed maternal world to the world of relationship and social exchanges. In the same way as the cocoon of the silk worm must be pierced to allow a new form to emerge, something must pierce the maternal world to allow for the meta-morphosis of the subjective.

But, if the 'phallus' in this way makes a hole in the maternal world, it is as the result of a displacement of the maternal desire towards it: from an exaggerated and self-sufficient form (the great phallus of the erect biped: see above) it becomes the external genital object which is the penis. But the penis is not just a kind of miniature bonsai of the erect body; it is the expression of the incompleteness of the mother's body and the figurative representation of otherness.

In the end, the phallus constitutes the primordial symbolic object only because its relationship to the mother–child dyad is external. In other words, it is the desire of the mother for the phallus which introduces it into the original relation, in a metaphoric way. The original symbolic instance is thus engraved at the very centre of the maternal world, the mark of an irreparable loss of completeness. The recognition of this incompleteness signifies the abandonment, more or less abrupt or progressive, of magical thought, in favour of a more realistic acceptance of the non-personal dimensions of the environment.

For all that, the primordial matrices of the imaginary are not simply discarded like waste products in the subjective adventure. Rather, the imaginary is recruited to serve in more abstract representations, in the symbolic agencies which rule the social order and in the design of the relations between the sexes, between the ages and generations, and between the clans and classes. On this point, Lacan clearly refers to an extensive vision which, far from reducing the phallus to a purely sexual connotation, is aimed at releasing psychoanalysis from the narrow limits of the individual psyche:

> the slightest alteration in the relation between man and the signifier . . . changes the whole course of history by modifying the moorings that anchor his being. It is precisely in this that Freudianism, however misunderstood it has been, and however confused its consequences have been, to anyone capable of perceiving the changes we have lived through in our own lives, is seen to have founded an intangible but radical revolution. (Lacan, 1977: 174)

To illustrate the affinity of Lacan's inspiration with what he called the 'science of marriage', one can turn to the article Lévi-Strauss wrote in homage to Josselin de Jong, entitled 'Do dual organizations exist?' In this article, Lévi-Strauss first comments on the extraordinarily wide distribution of dual systems around the world, but he emphasises at the same time that 'the relation between the moieties is never as static nor as reciprocal as one might tend to imagine' (1963: 135). Starting with Malinowski's description of the village of Omarakana and those of Geise in Java and others, he shows, in effect, how the division into moieties is itself cut through by an opposition of another kind, between the central (sacred) and peripheral (profane). In the Bororo village, one sees how a dualist exogamy (affecting the clans) exists alongside a triadic endogamy, resulting from the superimposition of three classes (high, middle, low). These observations, presented here in a very abridged form, call into question a simple application of the theory of reciprocity to explain such dual organisation, and which must then explain away irregularities in terms of historical contingency or other factors. Lévi-Strauss, on the contrary, sets out to show that if one gives up the illusion of a pure dualism, an extra dimension clearly emerges: 'If we treat in terms of ternary systems those forms of social organization which are usually described as binary, their anomalies vanish, and it then becomes possible to reduce them all to the same type of formalization' (Lévi-Strauss, 1963: 154).

In brief, a third element must interpose itself in order to materialise a metaphoric dimension in the social body and in the local cosmology. This is the same conclusion to the dialectic of forms as that reached from a study of the process of the development of subjectivity. The dimensions high–low, sacred–profane, etc., are no more artefacts coming to disturb the egalitarian harmony of exchanges than the symbolic agency is for the subject. Rather, they appear, in the historical conditions of these societies, as the principle of obligatory return in the practice of reciprocity.

Let me finish my commentary by conjuring up an image which, I hope, will not be found to be too outrageously patriotic for this Franco-British collaboration. I want to talk of the Concorde: not the aeroplane but the place of the same name. It takes, as one knows, the form of an octagon, with an obelisk marking the centre and each corner occupied by a plinth surmounted by a status of a woman, representing a town found, more or less, at the boundaries of the national territory. In fact, this obelisk is the third occupant of the centre. Originally, the present 'Concorde' was the royal square and had a golden statue of Louis XV at its centre. In 1792, this equestrian statue was melted down and a stately 'Liberty', made by Lemot, was installed at the centre of what had become the 'Square of the Revolution'. It was at the foot of this modern divinity that the guillotine was placed. When the bourgeois power decided to remove such vestiges of that troubled period from memory, the square was given its present name and an obelisk was installed there in 1838.

So, we have three central figures for the three segments of the national history. There is much to say of this series of three fetishes but we will content ourselves with the plan of the most recent, the present Concorde. Seen from the centre, the square appears as a succession of long perspectives, parting as rays from the statues of the women/towns. The millions of tourists who pass by can legitimately see in them a somewhat naughty evocation of the French spirit.

It is not necessary to be a psychoanalyst to notice a sexual dimension in the composition, in which a stone phallus is the candle at the centre of a circle of matrons who seem to cast a proprietorial regard over it. From this point of view, the message is simple and can be briefly summarised in this way: the political centre is as necessary to the distant provinces as the idea that strikes men that it is the incompleteness of women which transforms their own genitalia into the desirable phallus.

What is important to grasp here is the particular quality of the ideology presented in this way. On the one side, there is in this scenario an ideal fusion between the provinces and the centre, a fantasy of a glorious copulation of forms which could be the basis of national unity. On the other side, there are the grand centrifugal perspectives, with the whole producing a pulsating effect, an impression of permanence which makes play with the tension between the far and the near and which reunites the categories of self and other.

However, the crossroads has evolved down the course of the centuries to become an extremely complex web. One axis links the church of the Madeleine to the Bourbon Palace, which, despite its name, is the symbol of republican power. This is crossed by a second axis, Louvre – Arche de la Défense. This route links the cultural pole (extending towards the East as far as the Opera Bastille and the project for a new National Library) to the economic seat of power (found in the west), and passing through the military axis of the Arc de Triomphe and the Avenue de la Grande Armée. This route does more than span a distance, it also concerns a temporal journey, from the feudal roots of the nation (the Château de Philippe Auguste exhibited in the underground room of the Louvre is the most remarkable example) to the futurism of the towers of the Défense, with the Arche de la Defénse at the apex. It is the furthermost point in the perspective, but its size is so colossal that the distance seems to disappear (in fact, it does not seem any further away than the Arc de Triomphe, despite the several kilometres between them) so that it seems to provoke an inversion of the centrifugal effect.

To conclude, I hope that I have contributed some elements to suggest the idea of a short-circuit between the phallocentric moment in which the human person is structured and the relations of domination in society. As in the example, one sees fantasy made into a political fable in which the sexual speaks the language of the social order and follows its rhetoric in all its complexity. Nothing is simple.

BIBLIOGRAPHY

Lacan, J. (1977) *Ecrits: A Selection*, trans. A. Sheridan. London: Tavistock.
Lévi-Strauss, C. (1963) 'Do dual organizations exist?', in *Structural Anthropology*. Harmondsworth: Penguin.

Part IV
Working models

11 Indulgent fathers and collective male violence

L. R. Hiatt

Towards the end of an essay I published a few years ago on 'Freud and anthropology' (Hiatt, 1987), I made some tentative remarks about the Oedipus complex in the light of modern studies in behavioural primatology and brain evolution. More recently, I attempted to develop this perspective in an article called 'Towards a natural history of fatherhood' (Hiatt, 1990). The present paper continues the project by examining the relationship between fathers and sons in the context of initiation among the Australian Aborigines. The empirical materials are drawn largely from *On Aboriginal Religion* by W. E. H. Stanner, published first as a series of articles in Oceania between 1959 and 1963 and later as a monograph.[1] However, I touch on a more general issue, viz. what is the significance for psycho-analytic theory of the fact that fathers in many cultures not only love their sons but behave lovingly towards them?

As we all know, the archetypal father of *Totem and Taboo* was a violent male who defended his harem against all-comers and expelled his sons from the primal horde as they reached maturity. Freud based his depiction on some speculations by Darwin about early human breeding units, as well as certain statements by Atkinson concerning 'parricide' in herds of wild cattle and horses (Freud, 1919: 325). However, we learn virtually nothing about the primal sire except that he had a bad temper. The representation of the sons is more complex: as well as hostility for the father, they also felt tenderness, and hence remorse for their rebellion against him. Why they should have been fond of the tyrant who made lives miserable remains a mystery. One looks in vain for a mention of paternal love.

The contrast between Freudian archetype and anthropological reality is stark. In the ethnographic record, paternal love abounds. The implication of this fact for psychoanalytic theory was discussed incisively by Spiro in his important book *Oedipus in the Trobriands* (1982). More recently, Hewlett (1991) has presented the most systematic account of paternal love among hunter-gatherers yet published. In his book *Intimate Fathers* he says that among Aka Pygmies of the Congo fathers nurse infants almost half as much as their mothers do, and are more likely than the latter to hug, kiss or clean them. They effectively soothe infants by singing softly and humming. Infants seek proximity to their fathers about half as frequently as to their mothers, and more frequently than to all other individuals combined. Aka mothers are more likely than fathers to become angry with offspring and to rebuke or punish them for naughtiness.

Annette Hamilton's book on Aboriginal child-rearing in Arnhem Land (Hamilton, 1981) tells a similar story, though Aboriginal fathers are perhaps not such conscientious nursers as their Aka counterparts. For the first 18 months of its life, an infant is in intensive physical contact with its biological mother. The father's interaction increases from about 6 months, though only in verbal communication. Interestingly, while mothers rebuke their offspring (often using obscenities), fathers never do. (In fact men in my experience are prone to remonstrate with their wives for unnecessary harshness.) Hamilton formed an impression 'of children living in a highly emotional world with their mothers while "sensible" rational exchanges take place with fathers and other men' (1981: 63). From the age of about 3 years, boys move increasingly towards their fathers, whose tolerance of their demands for attention is nothing short of remarkable. They are given no codes of behaviour, taught no moral laws and given virtually no discipline. From the age of about 5 years until puberty they run wild with their peers, though they also associate with their fathers and older brothers, especially if they are doing something interesting.

It is possible that the above two examples are not representative. Nevertheless, I am confident that if we were to construct a portrait of the father in hunting and gathering societies from all the data available, it would bear a much closer resemblance to the fathers described by Hewlett and Hamilton than to the primal sire sketched by Freud. Although we are not bound to assume that the paradigm father among contemporary or recent hunters provides the best evidence for speculating about the archetypal father in remote antiquity, radical differences between the two models would be discouraging.

Freud subsequently came much closer to ethnographic realities in *Civilization and its Discontents*, where he suggested that the human family has its origins in the loss of oestrus and continuous sexual receptivity in the female. This, he thought, gave the male an incentive for keeping the female near him. The female, for her part, stayed near the male so that her helpless young would be provided with added protection. However it came about, concealed ovulation established new conditions for male reproductive success (Alexander and Noonan, 1979; Turke, 1984). Normally among the social primates the optimal male strategy is to seek exclusive access to as many females as possible at the peak of oestrus. Male parental care of individual offspring is rare. But once it becomes difficult if not impossible to discern whether females are ovulating or not, the chance of achieving fertilisation through any particular copulatory act becomes random. Males come under selective pressure to spend greater lengths of time with smaller numbers of females. The reproductive success of a particular male, in other words, becomes correlated with prolongation of sexual activity with a particular female, combined with simultaneous reduction of access to her by other males. Sexual selection of males by females is correspondingly accorded more favourable conditions in which to operate, and female reproductive interests dictate a preference for males with child-rearing proclivities.

If this view is correct, it would imply that caring fathers have been in existence for a long time in the human species, and it would also help to explain why their occurrence ethnographically is so widespread. It should be added that, as far as one can judge from overt behaviour, paternal affection is generally reciprocated. Filial love is commonplace, though, of course, not necessarily unqualified.

In Australia, perhaps nowhere is the solicitude of fathers more in evidence than during the initiation of their sons at puberty. Among the Aranda, the foreskin of the circumcised lad is pressed against the belly of the father and older brother to soften the pain they felt during the operation.[2] Stanner notes that among the Murinbata paternal anxiety reaches a peak as men form a cluster around the novice and shout loudly to drown his cries:

> It is at this instant that spear-throwing is most likely. On one occasion Ngunima, a particularly fierce man of the Kutjil clan, beside himself with sorrow and anger about the suffering of Dapan, his adopted son, killed the boy's mother with one spear and with another pierced the surgeon through both legs. A third spear wounded another woman. True to his craft, the surgeon went on to complete the operation. Ngunima was later called to account but survived the battle. (Stanner, 1989: 116, fn.12)

This, I think, would have to be a unique case. Normally, fathers control whatever anguish they may feel during the operation and swell with pride once their sons have come bravely through it. Nevertheless, the position of the father is felt to be an awkward one, and in many tribes institutionalised structural arrangements exist for the purpose of easing some of the attendant tensions. The general effect is to distance the father from any appearance of personal responsibility for what is happening. Even though his formal consent is required before initiation procedures can be set in motion, his subsequent role is entirely passive. All actions likely to cause distress to the boy and his family, particularly his mother and female kin, are carried out by designated others. In at least one tribe, the Tiwi of Bathurst and Melville Islands, the father even feigns surprise at events he himself has helped to pre-arrange.

> Though the father instigated and stage managed the whole affair, he and his household were always thunderstruck when the cross-cousins – armed to the teeth and painted like a war party – arrived at his camp one evening and proceeded to carry off forcibly the yelling 14-year-old. He had to be dragged literally from the bosom of his family, with his mother screaming and trying to hide him and the father pretending to resist the invaders of his household. From then on, until the final stage . . . at age 24–26, the boy was completely under the authority of the men who carried him off. (Hart, Pilling and Goodale, 1988: 103)

Sometime in the early 1950s Stanner drafted a brief polemic against *Totem and Taboo*, which he apparently never sought to publish and which appeared in print only after his death (Stanner, 1982). The object of the critique was to demonstrate that Freud's reading of the Oedipus myth is distorted and misleading, and more generally that his understanding of human social relationships is fallacious. About the same time Stanner was working on the corpus of myth and rite that later formed the empirical core of his monograph (1989). This includes the myth of the Rainbow Serpent as he recorded it among the Murinbata of Port Keats (Northern Territory). The central characters are Kunmanggur (the Rainbow Serpent), his two daughters (Green Parrots) and his son Tjiniman (the Bat). The transcript runs to several thousand words (1989: 88–94); here I paraphrase and reduce it to its main narrative elements.

> One day Kunmanggur's pubescent daughters set out on a food-gathering expedition. 'Father', they said,'we are going that way, to look for food.'
> Tjiniman, who had just been circumcised and whose penis was still painful, saw them and followed. On observing traces of menstrual blood where they had rested, he became sexually excited. When he overtook the girls, he displayed an erection and ejaculated.
> That evening he went for a walk. He removed his pubic covering, and hornets stung his penis so that it swelled enormously. After dark he returned and proposed intercourse. The girls indignantly refused, reminding him that they were his sisters. He threatened them with sorcery, and they submitted to a brutal rape that continued throughout the night. The following day the two sisters escaped and later enticed Tjiniman to climb after them up a cliff face by rope. As he neared the top, they severed the rope and he fell onto the rocks below, breaking many bones. By magical means he repaired his injuries and had a good sleep.

When he woke up he flaked a stone and tried to cut his nose. The instrument was too blunt. He tried more flakes and eventually found one that cut sharply through his nose. He magically repaired the wound.

Then he returned home. A day later he told his father he was going to a place where bamboo grows in order to make himself a spear. Before leaving he complained to a 'brother-in-law' about the injuries he had suffered. 'No one looked after me', he said, 'I fell down on the stones.'

After making a spear, he visited many people and invited them to a dance in honour of his father ('the Old One', 'the Leader-Friend'). He led them back to his father's home, making smoke signals from the hill tops on the way back. His father welcomed him.

'What news?' he asked. 'Many people are coming to dance,' Tjiniman replied.

The dancing began. Kunmanggur played the didjeridu. His two daughters had told him about the rape. They sat near him. Tjiniman danced vigorously, to make women desire him. The noise and excitement grew. Then Tjiniman said in a language no one understood: 'I am going to kill your father.' This he repeated several times. At length the singers began the last song. As Kunmanggur blew into the didjeridu, Tjiniman came close and plunged his spear into his father's back.

The Old One rolled about in agony. Tjiniman fled, and, standing far off, looked back and wondered what the people would do. But no one took revenge.

Kunmanggur died slowly, leaving behind manifestations of himself in the landscape that are still visible today. Nearing the end, and feeling weary and angry, he gathered all the fire and placed it on his head like a head-dress. As he walked into the sea, someone cried out that he intended to extinguish it. Pilirin (the Kestrel) tried to snatch it from him, but too late. It was out. Pilirin then showed men for the first time how to use fire drills.

Kunmanggur thrashed about in the water and then sank from sight. Where he went down is now called 'Place of the Great Mother'.

When Stanner first presented a summary of this myth to a public audience in 1958, he said: 'A book could be written – indeed, I cannot promise not to write it – about the symbolisms of the myth' (1979: 55). Although the thought never quite fathered the deed, some of the interpretative sections of *On Aboriginal Religion* indicate the main direction such a book would have taken. We can be sure Freud would not have figured largely in it. Having summarily dismissed *Totem and Taboo* as the product of misguided genius, Stanner in his working paper had effectively cleared the way for himself to ignore ontogeny and discover in the primal parricide of Kunmanggur a hidden ontology.

The presentation of the myth is followed by an attempt to contextualise it on the basis of native exegesis and comment. Although not linked with an extant ritual, it 'impinged rather more widely and deeply on the mystical beliefs of the Murinbata than any other' (1979: 95). Kunmanggur was represented as a beneficent culture hero, a great man of superhuman size and powers, the creator of humankind. In some statements there were suggestions that he was linked somehow with a female creator ('the Oldest Woman'), or even that Kunmanggur was bisexual. After dying, he was transformed into a serpent with a scorpion-like tail, who lives in the deep and appears from time to time in the form of the rainbow.

Before making his interpretative 'leap in the dark', Stanner wrote a preamble that might conceivably have been intended as a taunt to Freudians in the manner of Nabokov.

> For here is a myth standing alone as though it were a monument to something forgotten but vaguely familiar, and rife with suggestive silences. . . . From what motive did [Tjiniman] go on to heal, mutilate and again heal himself? And then seek his father's death? . . . The son's animus towards his father, and the father's intent towards the son, are left dark. . . . And, among the aborigines who are alive, Tjiniman is not execrated and Kunmanggur not mourned: all one can detect is a certain amusement about the memory of one and a certain warmth about the memory of the other. (Stanner, 1989: 100)

Having left these and other questions hanging in the air, Stanner makes a structural comparison between the Rainbow Serpent myth and two other 'dramas' (the bullroarer rite and its associated myth) discussed earlier in the monograph. He finds them to be homomorphic. Through their common structure they express a certain view about the nature of existence, an ontology that permeates Murinbata religious theory and practice. Murinbata religion, according to Stanner, is 'the celebration of a dependent life which is conceived as having taken a wrongful turn at the beginning, a turn such that the good life is now inseparably connected with suffering' (1989: 39). Some unexplained primal malfeasance has bequeathed to humans a life of qualified goodness, a flawed sociality where security is undermined by latent treachery and joy coexists with suffering. At the centre of things social, refuge and rottenness are found together. Murinbata ontology expresses an intuition of an integral moral flaw in human association (1989: 44).

It is interesting to compare this formulation of the Murinbata philosophy with Stanner's summary characterisation of Freudian psychology, which he finds cynical, distasteful and misconceived: a view of 'relations flawed through and through by ambivalence, domination, illusion, imbalance, instability, frustration, infantilism' (1982: 7). In fact, the homology between Murinbata ontology and Freudian ontogeny would be quite impressive. An idyllic period at the beginning of history, corrupted by a mysterious act of betrayal, and in consequence life as we now know it = pre-Oedipal bliss, the primal scene and the ensuing struggle between the pleasure and reality principles. Murinbata mythology in that case would be an ontological superstructure erected on an Oedipal base.

This is an interesting possibility, which I have considered elsewhere (Hiatt, 1975, 1989). Here, however, I should like to proceed by making a closer examination of the Rainbow Serpent myth. The central character, in terms of dramatic development, is Tjiniman. He is present from the beginning until almost the end, and his desires and actions give the narrative its shape. The myth, we may therefore presume, expresses the perspective of the Son rather than the Father.[3]

When the drama begins, Tjiniman is a young man experiencing the post-operative pain of circumcision. Simultaneously he lusts for his sisters. The conjunction may not be accidental. Among the Murinbata, so we are told, boys experiment sexually with their clan-sisters before puberty; immediately after circumcision they are warned by senior men that, although they are now eligible for sexual relationships, they should on no account have anything to do with their clan-sisters (Falkenberg, 1981: 77–9). Circumcision may be conceived as a warning against incest in the future and possibly as a punishment for transgressions in the past.

The motif of incestuous desire (or incest itself) followed by injury and pain is repeated several times. Tjiniman removes his pubic covering as a prelude to raping his sisters, and hornets sting his penis. After the rape, they sting him again. When he climbs up a rope towards his sisters (a variation on displaying an erection to them?), they cut the rope and he falls to the ground.

From this point Tjiniman becomes increasingly autonomous in dealing with his desires and sufferings. He repairs his broken bones; then, as though to prove a point, he cuts his own nose (penis?) and magically restores it. Subsequently he tells a friend, related to him as an affine: 'No one looked after me.' Perhaps he means: 'I was prevented from satisfying my desires. My own family has rejected [ejected?] me.' After one last attempt to excite his sisters (by dancing), he kills Kunmanggur and leaves. The Father, kind and benevolent though he is, pays the penalty for the frustration and punishment of the incestuous longings of the Son. No one avenges this awesome patricide. In the morality of the unconscious, the act is justified.

Stanner recorded fragmentary versions of the Rainbow Serpent myth in three neighbouring tribes. None appears to involve patricide. The Nangiomeri variant is the most coherent.

Angamunggi, the Rainbow Serpent, is the primeval Father, the maker of spirit-children, and the protector of humankind. Although male, he has a womb and once gave birth to a son who died and now forms a section of the rainbow.

Adirminmin, the Flying Fox, was married to two of the Rainbow Serpent's sisters. He made a spear and went hunting. His two wives hid from him, then called from the top of a cliff. They lowered a rope, which broke as he ascended. He fell and broke many bones, which he mended himself.

The two sisters ran back to the Rainbow Serpent, with sexual intent. Flying Fox pursued them across a river, but the tide kept sweeping him back. He found a sharp stone and made a spear. At length he overtook his wives. He sang a song and danced by himself. Afterwards he slept. Waking, he found the Rainbow Serpent and speared him in the back. (Stanner, 1989: 87–8)

We see here an interesting inversion. In the Murinbata myth an incestuous man is injured while pursuing his sisters and then kills his father. In the Nangiomeri myth, a married man is injured while pursuing his incestuous wives and then kills their brother. We might be inclined to infer that in some sense both myths are concerned with sibling incest and its repudiation. Let us explore this theme further in the context of initiation ritual.

To achieve full manhood, a Murinbata boy must pass through three rituals: a pre-puberty rite, circumcision and the bullroarer rite.

PRE-PUBERTY RITE

The night before the ceremony begins, the novices sleep together in the centre of the camp-circle. The following morning they are taken by the men into the bush to the ceremonial ground, where they are placed under the guardianship of their brothers-in-law.

From now on they are referred to as 'dingoes' (native dogs) and placed under a speech taboo. Boys thought to be in need of discipline are forced to lie face up in the sun with their eyes open.

The next seven days are occupied with singing and dancing.

Then most of the men disappear. One of the guardians explains to the novices that they have gone to prepare for a fight. Pretending to be concerned for their safety, he leads them back towards the main camp. They notice fires burning close to the path.

Suddenly masked men leap from hiding, grunting ominously and hurling weapons. In fear of their lives, the novices run wildly back to the ceremonial ground where, on arriving safely, they are given fire-drills by their brothers-in-law.

The next day the boys are decorated by their brothers-in-law and taken back to their families in the general camp. For another month they must remain silent in the presence of their female kin. Then gifts of food are made to their brothers-in-law, cooked on fires lit by the fire-drills they received at the ceremonial ground.

CIRCUMCISION RITE

On a pre-arranged day, people gather at the camp of the boy's father. Close relatives form a cluster in the centre, while singers, musicians and dancers perform for several hours. On cue, the music stops abruptly and a future wife's brother of the novice steps forward, places a hand on the lad's shoulder, and says: 'Now I take you to make you a man.' Amidst wailing and self-mutilation, the boy is led away by his affine from the cluster of close kin.

The brother-in-law takes the boy on a tour of neighbouring and distant communities, accompanied by singers and dancers. The journey might last several months, during which the novice enjoys the excitement of seeing new places and people. At the same time he is subject to new disciplines, including food taboos and obedience to his guardians and mentors.

The escort party dramatically announces its return by throwing a ceremonial spear into the centre of the home community's circle of camp-fires. At the sight of the white tuft quivering in the firelight, the boy's close kin give forth with lamentations.

On the afternoon of the next day, following a morning of growing excitement, a long line of decorated men appears about 500 metres away, heading towards the main camp. After a series of advances and retreats, they bring the novice to within 50 metres of his close kin. Weeping profusely, the latter rush forward and attempt to wrest the lad away from his guardians.

The men interpose themselves between the boy and his mother, and form a dense screen around the novice. Four of his classificatory brothers-in-law interlace their legs to make a platform on which the boy is placed and held while a surgeon removes his foreskin.

For several weeks the circumcised youth stays in the care of his brother-in-law, though food is provided by his mother. Then he is ritually cleansed and decorated.

BULLROARER RITE

This rite, known as Punj, inducts circumcised youths into the cult of the Mother. It occurs annually and lasts a month or so.[4]

The postulants are led by a senior man to a secret clearing. Initiated adult males have already assembled. When the youths arrive, the initiates enclose them in a tight circle. They sing a psalm which ends with an invocation of the Mother. The men return with the novices to the main camp, where the latter sit in a position of honour.

Before dawn the next day, the lads return to the ceremonial ground. The morning begins with a playful exchange of obscenities between men related as classificatory affines, then is taken up with singing. In the early afternoon, the novices are told to remove their clothing and orna- ments. From now on they are referred to as 'dingoes', and their personal names are not used. They are informed that soon the Mother will arrive and swallow them alive, then vomit them up.

The initiates perform the mime of the blowfly, making small agitated movements and a low-pitched buzzing sound. The postulants are then covered with blood, which they are told comes from the Mother but which actually comes from the veins of their future wives' brothers. Then they hear the sound of the bullroarers, said to be the voice of the Mother. As the sound comes closer, and the initiates simulate fear, the novices prepare for the worst. Suddenly men swinging the bullroarers leap into view. Brothers- in-law of the novices come forward, each bearing a bullroarer covered with his own blood, which he thrusts between the thighs of his sister's future husband at the angle of an erect penis.

Each day, from now until the end of the ceremony, proceedings follow a regular pattern: singing in a tight circle, ritual obscenities, the mime of the blowfly, songs and dances celebrating totemic ancestors. On the final day youths are anointed with blood and presented with gifts by their brothers-in-law. All the men proceed to the main camp, where the novices' female kin have been assembled. The men form two long lines. On a signal from the elders, the youths emerge from concealment and crawl through the tunnels formed by the men's outspread legs. On emerging, each youth sits momentarily in front of his mother, with his back to her, but not touching or touched by her, while the women wail and lacerate their heads. The lads then return through the tunnel of legs, and all the men rush back to the ceremonial ground.

A week after the end of the ceremony, the youths bathe and have a cryptic insignia of the bullroarer painted on their bodies. They return to the main camp to resume normal life, except that from now on they must not go near their mothers' hearths. After a couple of years, they are judged to be ready for marriage.

If the Rainbow Serpent myths presented above are concerned primarily with sibling incest, the initiation rites seem directed rather more to the repudiation of mothers. Throughout Australia, when lads are formally removed from their family circles, it is understood that the separation is primarily of sons from mothers.[5] This would seem to be the point of the Murinbata designation of novices as 'dingoes'; in the whelping season, men take dingo pups from their mothers in order to tame them. When a boy is about to be circumcised, men interpose themselves between him and his mother, who is shouldered aside (Stanner 1989: 115). At the end of the bullroarer rite, the newly inducted youths go to their mothers in order to turn their backs on them.

The universal Mother from whom the lads have been delivered, so that they may become men, is an ancestral cannibal named Karwadi. The following myth is central to the bullroarer cult:

The people decided to go on a honey-foraging expedition. Before setting out, they asked Karwadi to take care of the children. After bathing in the river, the children gathered around their minder. On the pretext of delousing them, Karwadi picked them up one by one and swallowed them, then fled.

The parents returned and realised what had happened. The men set out in pursuit and overtook Karwadi as she crawled underwater along a creek bed. A man called Left Hand speared her through the legs, while another called Right Hand broke her neck with a club. When they cut open her belly, they found the children alive and well in her womb. The two men lifted them out, washed and adorned them, then returned them to their mothers. (Stanner, 1989: 40–2)

In commenting on this myth, Stanner remarks that the devouring Mother has to be killed as 'the condition of the perpetuation of human life through its children' (1989: 80). This is an inference from native exegesis, not an application of psychoanalytic theory. Each day in the Punj ceremony, men emit the humming sound of the blowfly inside an excavation symbolising the Mother. As the association is with rotting flesh (1989: 7), we may presume that the mime signifies her death. When her power is climactically revealed as an artefact manipulated by initiated men, each youth receives the gift of an erect bullroarer between his thighs. The dissolution of links with the Mother's flesh is simultaneously a condition of sexual potency and admission to the male domain of the spirit.

In an account of totemic ceremonies among the Aranda of Central Australia, T. G. H. Strehlow concludes that:

the great mystery revealed to the human totemites in the final acts of their ceremonial cycles was the eternal union, in an unbreakable embrace, of the separate male and female 'principles' which had always co-existed at each sacred site. (Strehlow, 1964: 738)

The applicability of the statement goes far beyond the Aranda, even if it is not true of male secret cults everywhere in Australia. We may therefore frame an apparently curious question. Why is it that junior males are formally separated from their mothers so that they may witness in the secret company of senior males, including their fathers, a recapitulation of the primal act of sexual union?

Many observers have noted the camaraderie that pervades cult life among Aborigines, manifest in ribaldry, good humour, co-operation, singing and moving in unison, high levels of body contact and periodic euphoria. Once novices have endured the pain and humiliation of initiation, they enter a domain of mateship and equality. Conflict and argument are formally banned from the ceremonial precinct. If necessary, opportunities are provided for men to settle their grievances before the rituals begin. Peacefulness and the exclusion of females are thus regarded by Aboriginal men as necessary conditions of the highest forms of the religious life; and, given what we know of the main causes of trouble in daily life, we may assume that the first is not unconnected in their minds with the second.

The evidence we have been considering strongly suggests that the *primal* grievance between males is settled, not before the ceremony begins, but in the ceremony itself. In those cases where the climax is the revelation of the primal act of sexual union, there is a sense in which it might be true to say that the underlying purpose of the ritual is to resolve the primal flaw in the relationship between father and son by exposing its nature and dramatising its cause as the common fate of all men. Through the agency of collective male violence, a youth's libido is detached from his mother and sisters and steered towards his future wife. At the same time love for his father is preserved and strengthened by the cathartic dissipation of residues of Oedipal resentment. From this firm platform, underpinned by already established associations with boyhood age-mates, each youth is launched into the world of men.

NOTES

1 In so doing, I pay homage to Stanner as a great Australian ethnographer and thank Oceania Publications for allowing me to reproduce his data. I am grateful to the same publisher for permission to use material from my introduction to the 1989 edition of the monograph.
2 Reported by Carl Strehlow in his monograph *Die Aranda- und Loritja-Staemme in Zentral Australien, 1907-21*. I am grateful to Hans Oberscheidt for allowing me to read in manuscript his forthcoming English translation.
3 During the 1950s a nativistic cult arose in the East Kimberley region of Western Australia, in which Jesus was referred to as Tjiniman.
4 It is possible that the Murinbata Rainbow Serpent myth was once connected with a secret cult. In any event, we recall that, as the Father dies, he descends

into the Place of the Mother. Whether this represents eternal union of male and female principles is open to speculation.

5 Hamilton (1981: 68) reports the case of a 7-year-old lad who refused to give up his mother's breast. In the event, he was seized by adult males and circumcised.

BIBLIOGRAPHY

Alexander, R. and Noonan, K. (1979) 'Concealment of ovulation, parental care and human social evolution', in N. Chagnon and W. Irons (eds) *Evolutionary Biology and Human Social Behavior*. North Scituate: Duxbury.

Falkenberg, A. and Falkenberg, J. (1981) *The Affinal Relationship System: A New Approach to Kinship and Marriage among the Australian Aborigines at Port Keats*. Oslo: Universitetsforlaget.

Freud, S. (1919) *Totem and Taboo*. New York: Moffat, Yard.

—— (1963) *Civilisation and its Discontents. S.E.* 21.

Hamilton, A. (1981) *Nature and Nurture*. Canberra: Australian Institute of Aboriginal Studies.

Hart, C., Pilling, A. and Goodale, J. (1988) *The Tiwi of North Australia*. New York: Holt, Rinehart & Winston.

Hewlett, B. (1991) *Intimate Fathers*. Ann Arbor: University of Michigan.

Hiatt, L. (1975) 'Introduction' to L. Hiatt (ed.) *Australian Aboriginal Mythology*. Canberra: Australian Institute of Aboriginal Studies.

—— (1987) 'Freud and anthropology', in D. Austin-Broos (ed.) *Creating Culture*. Sydney: Allen & Unwin.

—— (1989) 'Introduction' to W. Stanner, *On Aboriginal Religion*. Sydney: Oceania Publications.

—— (1990) 'Towards a natural history of fatherhood', *Australian Journal of Anthropology* 1: 110–30.

Spiro, M. (1982) *Oedipus in the Trobriands*. Chicago: Chicago University Press.

Stanner, W. (1979) *White Man Got No Dreaming*. Canberra: Australian National University Press.

—— (1982) 'On Freud's *Totem and Taboo*', *Canberra Anthropology* 5: 1–7.

—— (1989, originally 1959–63) *On Aboriginal Religion*. Sydney: Oceania Publications.

Strehlow, C. (1907–21) *Die Aranda- und Loritja-Staemme in Zentral Australien*. Frankfurt: Baer.

Strehlow, T. G. H. (1964) 'Personal monototemism in a polytotemic community', in *Festschrift für A.D. Jensen*. Munich: Klaus Renner Verlag.

Turke, P. (1984) 'Effects of ovulatory concealment and synchrony on protohominid mating systems and parental roles', *Ethnology and Sociobiology* 5: 33–44.

12 Every man a hero

Oedipal themes in Gisu circumcision[1]

Suzette Heald

How should an anthropologist use psychoanalysis? What can it add to our accounts? My starting position here is that it provides a hermeneutic which invites us to reinterrogate our data in order to both challenge and augment the interpretations already made on the basis of more standard forms of exegesis. In the Durkheimian tradition within which I have broadly worked, cultural values are taken to be relatively straightforwardly depicted in cultural symbolism. By contrast, psychoanalysis tells us that the symbolic process is complex, bedevilled by the forces of repression, whereby the manifest becomes a mask or, at best, a distorting mirror to psychic reality. If custom may be taken as symbolic in the psychoanalytic sense, speaking to unconscious fantasy and process, then it has the capacity to turn our accepted interpretative canons upside-down. In so doing, it does not, of course, invalidate the cultural interpretation. Devereux's postulate of 'complementarity' is useful here, though it is today less easy to see, as he did, that the coming together of the two perspectives will give a determinate understanding in either.

For many of us our first fieldwork proves the most formative experience of our lives and sets the agenda for much of what we do later. For me, it established a long-lasting source of intrigue with the topic of male circumcision. For the Gisu of Uganda, circumcision presents itself as a particularly severe ordeal which boys are required to undergo roughly between the ages of 17 and 25 in order to validate their claims to manhood. In previous writings, I have explored it from the point of view of what I called their 'vernacular psychology', how the Gisu see it as actually creating men, an identity forged in the ritual process (1982, 1989). In another paper (1986), I tried to trace the concordances of their view of this process with its transformational potential and western psychological theories, drawn largely from behaviourist psychology. In neither did I consider psychoanalysis. This is the challenge which I now take up and it is one which allows me to probe new areas, going beneath the overt level of culturally interpreted symbolism to look at how sexuality is encoded in the ritual. The challenge is, however, not without difficulties.

The first problem is epistemological. Anthropological commentary on psychoanalysis has frequently criticised it for its unprovable assumptions and analysis. For example, Leach castigates psychoanalysis for its 'atrocious techniques of hit or miss intuition' (1958: 149). This critique has always seemed inappropriate, as is the case when the pot calls the kettle black. As Cohen writes, 'psychoanalysis has at least as much claim to be considered a body of "scientific" ideas as do most others that are used by anthropologists in the study of symbolism' (1980: 48). Further, just as anthropology has reorientated its quest away from positivistic and natural science models of enquiry and towards more hermeneutic forms of understanding, so, too, a similar move has been argued for psychoanalysis. For Ricoeur (1979), Freud's true discovery lies in the realm of meaning, in the hermeneutics of suspicion, and thus in unravelling the deceptions of consciousness. The problems of validation of an interpretation are perhaps here no different from those that the anthropologist normally has to deal with; the unconscious dynamic must be shown to have some external correlative, either in the experience of the individual or in cultural practice. Nevertheless, whether in meaning or mechanism, the psychoanalytical model here frequently has an alternative mode of validation – which anthropology lacks – in its therapeutic claims. Thus, fantasy, symbol and ritual are deemed to have an observable effect on the emotional adjustment of individuals.

The second problem is to try to make sense of the claims made and to choose between rival readings of the 'theory'. Probably, the dominant line of argument relating to the practice of circumcision in the anthropological literature has its roots in Freud and the dynamics involved in the 'family romance', as he called it.[2] In the most general terms, circumcision has been seen as a response to ineffective repression of the Oedipal conflict in infancy. In adolescence, after the latency period, this has been seen to lead to a renewal of desire for the mother accompanied by hostile rivalry with the father. Further cultural buttresses are then seen as being required in order to solve the problems of psychic adjustment for individuals in these cultures, for example, by reinvoking castration anxiety through the practice of circumcision accompanied by taboos on sexual contact with senior women, taboos which have been seen as phobic responses to incest (see Reik, 1931, and, after him, Stephens and D'Andrade, 1962). The ritual then is seen to involve some kind of mimesis of the repressed conflicts encountered in childhood and the therapeutic dynamic is that of cathartic abreaction, serving to reconcile the son to his father's authority and to the cultural values which he represents and, most significantly, to the incest taboo.

In this context, Gisu circumcision presents itself initially as a striking negative example. It is an act which grants full adult status to a man and, in so doing, emancipates him from his father's authority. Further, there is no repression of antagonism. Indeed, circumcision marks the assumption of the most intense competition between father and son over the question of inheritance and this competition frequently results in violence. If we take manifest behaviour then, we cannot conclude the circumcision in this case effects the kind of reconciliation between father and son, a decrease in their rivalry, that we might expect.

How then should we read the theory? Do we conclude that the Oedipal conflict is either not universal or that resolution of it is not necessary? One problem here is that it is often not clear what 'resolution' means when anthropologists – or, indeed, psychoanalysts – invoke the concept. Is it, for example, a true resolution or does it involve further repression, with perhaps a new *modus vivendi*, but one equally liable to intra-psychic conflict? Further, if the process is largely unconscious, how are we to make the inferences we need for an evaluation? Unlike the psychoanalyst, the anthropologist has no transference material by which to validate his or her hypotheses. In part – but only in part – these problems arise from the type of causal developmental theory being used here, a theory which still sees culture as a 'psychic defence system', as Roheim (1934) put it, and which has not taken on the messages from more recent neo-Freudian work with its less deterministic framework. Psychoanalysis, like anthropology, has moved on and it is perhaps time to look at material such as initiation rites not so much as – or perhaps, not only as – being in the business of 'therapy' but as conveying messages about the way attachment to and detachment from the mother and resentment of the father may be handled in the particular cultural setting. If we take this as a starting point, it is apparent that the messages could be at variance with each other and may recapitulate conflicts without necessarily solving them. Ricoeur (1979, 1981) sees in Freud's genius not the pairing of symbol with a determinant meaning but the idea that the operations of fantasy betray no automatic laws, just as psychoanalysts find that individuals deal differently with reality and the defensive mechanisms they develop are labile and not fixed.

The choice in the interpretation of ritual then could be phrased as a choice between a developmental version which gives primacy to the formative experiences of childhood and sees ritual as emerging to solve these or a cultural account which gives priority to the ordering of symbolic meaning. In so far as this latter approach shifts the emphasis from the individual to culture it shifts the interpretation from a determinate psychodynamic developmental schema to a more variable one. Thus, the unconscious is seen as a resource which might be used to add emotive power to the ritual process and its dominant symbols, but without the implications of necessity. Among Africanists, it is well represented in the work of Fortes and Turner, both of whom managed to weld psychoanalytic insights into an otherwise Durkheimian perspective. For Durkheim, the key problem in social life was commitment and the role of religion was to galvanise both consciousness and conscience, impressing upon the individual the authority of culture and the supremacy of society. Fortes and Turner[3] both speculate upon how religion utilises the powers of the unconscious to this end, 'domesticating' conflicts, both intra-psychic and interpersonal. Further, Turner (1967) argues that, through the process of condensation, ritual symbols effect a synthesis of referents, drawing upon both emotionally charged physio-psychological processes and normative values. If this seems to give too much primacy to the social, with the idea that the resources of the *libido* are utilised for the purposes of social control, it nevertheless allows for a way of integrating the two perspectives, by emphasising not only the element of social control but also that of individual growth.

THEMES IN GISU CIRCUMCISION

If psychoanalytic understandings are to be used to inform cultural analysis, it is necessary first to outline briefly the dominant themes in Gisu circumcision and its emotional power.

The Gisu, who number some 500,000, are Bantu-speaking agriculturalists who live on the western slopes of Mount Elgon in Uganda. They lie at one end of a broad circumcising belt which runs down from Mount Elgon south and east through Kenya to Tanzania. Everywhere in this area, it would be fair to say, circumcision is strongly linked both to male gender identity and to ethnicity. Nowhere is this clearer than in Bugisu. The rituals of *imbalu* are held every two years during the month of August and the boys are required to stand upright for the operation betraying no signs of fear, pain or reluctance. As an ordeal, it thus has a critical personal dimension, an individual proof of masculinity, demonstrated in the courtyard of the boy's father or other senior relative and witnessed by an assembled throng of relatives and neighbours.

It is the ordeal which every young boy knows one day he must face and for which he has prepared himself by joining the circumcision parties for many years before he is finally ready to face the knife himself (to 'fall' or 'enter into' *imbalu*). When the time comes and he announces his decision, he is repeatedly told that he only has one chance – 'there is only one knife' – and that he should withdraw if he has any doubts rather than risk failure. Failure threatens on many counts, most evidently in the display of cowardice or fear which, in extreme cases, pollutes the circumcision knife and the compound of his father. But the whole of his adult life is also seen as dependent on *imbalu*. Much then is deemed at stake, but the emotional power of *imbalu* reaches far beyond this.

Undoubtedly, it is the most emotionally charged occasion for all Gisu men and, indeed, for the whole community, for whom its drama is re-enacted every two years. During the circumcision periods the whole of the countryside rings to the sound of the boys' bells and circumcision songs, and people are whipped up into states of intense excitement as they champion the candidates and urge them to bear it bravely. Dressed in the flamboyant regalia, the boys glory in the glamour of their position, the centre of everyone's attention and concern. Importantly, it is they who are seen as leading the country forward; it is their decision, their volition, their actions which mobilise their kin and their friends behind them. Further, in proving their manhood, they are in effect proving the identity of all Gisu as men and validating the power of the tradition which unites them all. 'Caught' by the ancestral power of circumcision, the boys, in effect, personify the power of the ancestors and the continuity of tradition.

Gisu circumcision is thus presented as a heroic act. Performed at a relatively late age when the boy is already physiologically and sexually mature, the rite can also explicitly be seen as a test of whether he is also, in Gisu terms, 'psychologically' a man, capable of demonstrating the force of character necessary to see the ritual through to completion. The key Gisu concept here is *lirima*, which in the present context can be glossed as 'anger'. The diacritical sign of *lirima* is however in the intensity of the emotion experienced. Thus it is spoken of as 'catching' a man or 'bubbling up' in him. While in this state of possession, *lirima* is seen to dictate all a man's attitudes and actions; it gives force to motivation and impels to action. In normal life *lirima* is linked to all the negative emotions, to jealousy, hatred, resentment and shame, and is seen as responsible for all the trouble in the community. It is only in circumcision that it is given a positive value. It *must* bubble up in the initiate so that all his actions are dominated by the overriding desire to see the ritual through to completion. If a man can be in the grip of *lirima* he can use it to steel himself too.

The intensity of *lirima*, its power and its 'bitterness' make this above all a manly attribute and women and boys are held not to experience it. They are held subject only to the lesser form of arousal of *libuba*. Circumcision thus becomes the first occasion on which a boy is required to display *lirima* and, as I have recounted elsewhere, this capacity then becomes as much a part of his manhood as the circumcision cuts themselves. Indeed, most of the symbolism of the preparatory ritual can be explicated in terms of the induction of *lirima* (Heald, 1982, 1986, 1989).

The linking of circumcision with the creation of *lirima* in the individual is central to the purposes of the rite. Having faced 'death' he is deemed free from the fear of it and capable of taking full responsibility for himself among other self-determining Gisu men. Indeed, circumcision is the first act of self-determination of a Gisu youth, transforming him from a mere boy, an appendage of his father, to a man, with a status equivalent to his father's. It is thus, above all, a rite of emancipation from parental authority and this has important political and economic correlates. After circumcision, a man is expected to marry and set up as an independent householder, responsible for providing for himself and for his own dependents. He is no longer reliant on his natal family for food, or even ritual protection, for he now becomes responsible for protecting his own family and may make sacrifices to the ancestors on his own behalf.

OEDIPAL ACCOUNTS: FATHER AND SON

Given this conscious frame for the interpretation of *imbalu*, it is difficult to tie it to the orthodox Freudian account of the significance of circumcision. Certainly, circumcision makes a son like his father; it clearly defines gender identity for the boy, removing him finally from the house of his mother and giving him the right to a wife and a house of his own. But arguments based on the classic account give a particular causal reading of this process which hinges on the recognition of the father's authority. It is fear of the father which motivates repression and the transference of desire and it is only in this context that circumcision has symbolic value as 'castration'. It makes circumcision an act of submission to the father and simultaneously to what he represents, the legitimate, if onerous, authority of culture represented in the incest taboo.

The whole tenor of the ritual argues against this. The rite is an act of emancipation and, in so far as one sees it as giving a very forceful stamp to male gender identity and the equivalence of all men, it is difficult to read it as an assertion of parental power.[4] Further, its themes offer a vivid contrast with many other initiation rituals. For example, Gisu boys are not passive initiates, dragged from the security of their homes to face unknown and terrifying ordeals in segregated ritual sites under the supervision of male elders. On the contrary, the ordeal is conceived of as an act of individual volition, with the boy freely choosing his year and thus making manifest the powers and capabilities of his ancestry. Indeed, the ritual exalts the act of individual choice and, in so doing, makes the son and not the father the vector of ancestral continuity. The locus begins and ends with the initiate himself, with the emphasis being upon the particular test of valour which it entails, a valour to which the Gisu give a particular interpretation and psychological meaning.

One way of saving circumcision for an Oedipal reading, however, would be to interpret it as a cultural fantasy serving to disguise the hidden reality of power in order to make it more palatable. But, to be plausible there must be tangible correlates in social arrangements which could be seen as motivating such a fantasy of weak paternal power. But, in Bugisu, parental authority is in reality weak and is accompanied by intense inter-generational conflict which frequently erupts into violence. Parricide is a real threat in Bugisu and so is filicide (La Fontaine, 1966; Heald, 1989). Nor can the operation be deemed to have therapeutic value as, for example, argued by Ottenberg for the Nigerian Afikpo, seeing it as 'an attempt to resolve psychological conflict between father and son, which serves to minimize (but not eliminate) frictions arising out of economic and political issues' (1988: 349). This it signally fails to do among the Gisu, for the attribution of violent power to both father and son in effect licenses the use of violence, which becomes a real possibility only after circumcision.

The problems at one level are all structural. After circumcision a father is obliged to provide for his son, that is, to begin to dismember his estate, allocating cattle for bridewealth to allow his son to marry and a parcel of land for him to farm and thus to feed himself and his wife. This obligation is considered absolute but is, in practice, often difficult to enforce. In the present situation of chronic land shortage, many men have insufficient land and run a serious risk of impoverishment by acceding to their sons' demands. Further, since every man is deemed an equal and in total control of his own affairs, such a distribution is in practice solely at the discretion of the father and no one has the right to intervene. Father and son are thus engaged in an essentially private dispute; one in which the son's rights are deemed absolute but can be enforced only by the son's own efforts at persuasion which, in the context, also include force.

The fact of circumcision then operates not to underplay competitive rivalry in the father and son relationship but to highlight it. Indeed, for both fathers and sons it creates a situation of double-bind. It establishes the son as an 'equal' but the essential economic resources he needs to establish himself as a full adult, that is, autonomous and self-sufficient, remain still with the father. Indeed, after a relatively free adolescence, circumcision brings to the fore this element of a boy's dependence. However, the way in which it does so serves not to ensure a son's subservience but to intensify the competitive element in their relationship by introducing the possibility of aggression. *Lirima* is deemed necessary for a man to defend his own interests against other men; the direct resort to physical force by the young or to witchcraft by the old is seen to follow from this. This is as likely in the father and son relationship as any other. Indeed, the nature of the com-petition between them makes it an added threat.

The ambivalence between father and son, seen as the core of the Oedipal complex by Freud, is thus not overcome by circumcision in any simple way. However, it may be seen to define the terms of the conflict dramatically, with the twin imperatives of the Oedipus complex – 'be like the father' (i.e., be a man like him) and 'don't be like the father' (i.e., don't take what is his, the mother) – reformulated in the contrast between aggression and sexuality. If the imperative 'to be like the father' is defined in terms of anger and autonomy – in effect, licensing competition – the imperative to be 'not like the father' is defined with respect to sexual prerogatives, outlawing competition in this particular sphere.

The generational divide with respect to sexuality and marriage in Bugisu is absolute. Women of the adjacent generation are totally prohibited and this includes both kinswomen and in-marrying affines. This rule clearly separates the sexual interests of fathers and sons.[5] At its simplest, women are divided into two major categories: those of the adjacent generation, whether kinswomen or affines, who are totally prohibited and those of one's own with whom one has a legitimate sexual interest. The generational patterning of sexual rights tends to override other distinctions in terms of consanguinity and sisters are, to this extent, substitute wives. This is clearly marked in the circumcision rituals.

Sisters – younger real sisters and also those of the kindred – accompany the boy during the last three days leading up to circumcision and are ritually smeared with millet yeast together with the boy. Later, again with the initiate, they are cleansed by the circumcisor after the operation and instructed on their role as future wives. At the time of first smearing, they are addressed as his 'wives' and this is usually explained in terms of the right a boy has to use some of their bridewealth in order to marry a wife of his own. While this applies most clearly to the boy's own younger sisters, it also applies by extension to more distant female kin since it is considered that marriages are contracted on behalf of the generation as a whole. These men may inherit each other's wives and compensation for adultery cannot be exacted. No such privileges are accorded between the generations. Thus, while all other forms of property are transmitted vertically, from seniors to juniors, sexual prerogatives are restricted to the generations, clearly demarcating the legitimate zones of interest for fathers and sons.

Fathers and sons may thus not compete sexually.[6] Indeed, the total opposition of the roles of mother and wife is a clear motif in Gisu life, and this finds expression in the way intimate relationships between the sexes are patterned. Women may only stand in one relationship to a man, either as a 'mother' or as a 'wife', and this is realised in particular taboos which restrict the breast to infants. Thus a man should not touch his wife's breasts and nor should she touch his genitalia for it is considered that that is a maternal role, for it is the mother who cleanses a man when he is young. Indeed, even when adult, if a man is ill and incontinent, it must be a woman related to him as a 'mother' who undertakes his physical care. Thus the Gisu are offered two possible but mutually incompatible models of conduct towards the opposite sex, that which one might call conjugal sexuality and the other, generative consanguinity.

If the transformation of desire from 'mothers' to 'sisters' is thus depicted in the ritual, this raises the question of how this effect might be achieved on a psychodynamic level. The mere picturing of the legitimate relationships, won through circumcision, though it forcefully expresses cultural propriety, raises the problem of how this is made palatable and how the ritual itself might be seen as aiding such a process. With this in mind, I now turn to the way in which sexuality is depicted in the rites.

SEXUAL SYMBOLISM

There are in fact few specifically sexual symbols at circumcision but, nevertheless, it is underwritten by a symbolism of process and powerful metaphors of sexuality and gestation run through it. These hinge on the symbolism of beer and fermentation. The whole ritual process is orchestrated with reference to the making of millet beer. The threshing of the millet for this beer is the first ritual act performed by the initiate and it is taken to signify intent. Later he initiates the last three-day fermentation cycle which leads up to his own circumcision by pouring water on the prepared millet and at the same time he is smeared from head to toe with millet yeast; the same yeast that is added to the brew. I have emphasised in previous accounts how this draws together two processes: the fermentation of beer and the development of *lirima* in the boy. The bubbling volatility of beer and its transformative powers provide a fitting metaphor for the fundamental nature of the change which the boy is deemed to be undergoing and this is directly linked to the growth of his 'anger'. But beer making also provides an important model by which the Gisu understand the process of gestation. Thus, pregnancy in women is likened to fermentation, with the 'white blood' of the man and the 'red blood' of the woman described as mixing together to form a child. Beer making thus exemplifies creative process, whether of fermentation, gestation and/or that involved in becoming a man.

In the course of the ritual attention is drawn to the similarity between these processes by a series of shouts. Firstly, as the boy pours the water on the beer, the shout goes up, 'You have spoilt it'. When he himself is circumcised, usually following the first cut, this is marked by the shout, 'They have spoilt you'. Lastly, one other event is marked in this way and that is when a girl is deflowered on her wedding night. Then it is said, 'He has spoilt you'. This constitutes an extended metaphor which can be unpacked in a number of ways.

In the first place, the word 'spoilt' is very definitely polysemic for the Gisu and carries a range of connotations. At one end it clearly designates our normal usage, something which has been subject to change and thus ruined: a useless thing. It is also applied to the spoiling of children through over-indulgence. Of the 'spoiling' at circumcision it may thus be said that the boy has been made useless and will not be able to engage in sexual intercourse or indeed in any normal life until he is finally cured. But at the other end of the scale, spoiling is seen as a necessary precondition for generative potential. Indeed, through the three shouts, explicit attention is being drawn to the parallels between circumcision, defloration and the adding of water to the brew. One idea that clearly links these occasions is the necessity for an original integrity of substance or persons to be destroyed in order for them later to fulfil their purpose. Water must be added to the millet before the yeast can activate fermentation; women must have their hymen ruptured before they can conceive and, likewise, a man should be cut before he can marry.

The spoiling is thus the necessary act for generation and such 'spoiling' is an achievement of culture. Women and men, no more than beer, are 'naturally' fertile: in all cases human agency has to work on the world of nature to release procreative potentiality and this destruction is performed culturally. The making of women is not more natural than the making of men or the making of beer. Or, to put it another way, natural fertility is created culturally, whether in people or in beer. One can also note that yeast, the generative agency in the case of beer, is also created culturally by germinating millet seeds. Again, when it sprouts, the millet is said to be spoilt. In all cases too, this is seen to lead to an increase in violence and aggressivity: the bubbling of the beer, the potency of a man linked to *lirima* and the turbulence created in the process of gestation which is held to explain the irritability of women during pregnancy.

At circumcision, the boy first 'spoils' the millet before himself becoming 'spoilt' and both acts carry the implications of sexuality. Indeed, the act of making beer is directly linked to sexuality and circumcision is the first time a boy participates in the task. Thereafter, when he marries, he will help his wife with the making of beer and when they do this they must abstain from sexual intercourse for the three days of the final fermentation lest the beer become 'too strong'. Beer brewing and sexuality are thus seen to interact positively as processes. With this in mind, we can explore further the significance of the boy making it together with his *mother* at circumcision.

MOTHER AND SON

Mother and son make the circumcision beer together, with the mother providing the millet and taking over from her son in completing all the tasks necessary for the final fermentation, including adding the yeast to the brew. In this, she may be seen as in actuality initiating the final fermentation after the, in a sense, false simulation of this when the boy pours the water on the millet. With beer making as a symbol of fertility and *lirima*, this makes the mother largely responsible for her son's courage just as it represents the mother rebirthing him. Indeed, this is clearly one implication. The mother's identification with her son is absolute and, daubing her face also with yeast, she may be symbolically seen to be going through a second birth of her son. This emerges clearly during the actual time of the operation when she retires to her house and takes up the attitude she had when giving birth, either standing or squatting, and often clasping the centre pole of her house.

Would it be too far-fetched to read the beer making as a representation of the libidinal bonds that bound the mother to her son in childhood? I think this might well be a valid interpretation, accompanied, as it is, with the substitution of wife for mother in the smearing ritual. One reading might be that, through her identification and 'rebirthing', the mother is symbolically releasing her son from his attachment to her and freeing him for independent adulthood. But, to give strength to this interpretation, we need to examine further the relationship of mother and son and take this back to infancy.

Since Freud, much psychoanalytic theory has come to emphasise the problems of separation and individuation and this has led to a re-evaluation of the mother and child relationship and the effects of early dependence. The relationship of this to the Oedipal complex itself is variously conceived but for many, including such diverse writers as Klein and Lacan, it involves the postulation of a pre-Oedipal situation in the fusion of the child with the mother in infancy. Childhood can be seen to involve a series of transitions as the child seeks to differentiate himself from the symbiotic union with the mother. For Lacan, the first relationship of a child with the mother is associated with what he calls the mirror phase. This constitutes the first step towards the realisation of subjectivity in the recognition which occurs around six months of age in an infant that he is a 'singular' entity. For Lacan, this is, as yet, an incomplete subjectivity which is only fully realised with the assumption of language when the subject takes on 'the dialectic of identification with the other', a stage which Lacan identifies with the Oedipal complex. The 'father' enters here as the destroyer of the mother/ child bond, a destruction necessary for the child to realise his own independent identity. The tangible effects of this for a child are maternal rejection and it is this which constitutes, for Lacan, the symbolic castration. As a universal predicament he postulates that the reaction to the loss must be repression. The desire for the mother is repudiated and made unconscious while the desire for the phallus is deferred.

If we are to look for the roots of individuation in early infancy, it is necessary to say more about this in the Gisu context. Unfortunately, I did not collect systematic data on post-partum sexual abstinence, age of weaning or mother–infant sleeping arrangements. Nevertheless, my observations lead me to suppose that weaning today is usually achieved around the end of the first year of life and that post-partum sexual taboos are often effectively lifted before the age of weaning. Weaning may be undertaken because of a new pregnancy or for fear of over-indulging the child. Thus a reason given for weaning is often that the child is becoming 'spoilt' and this fear gives a particular colouring to the process, with the child being reprimanded for his reliance on the breast. Here, fortunately, there is information of a kind not usually available to the anthropologist on the traumatic significance that such weaning may have.

THE JOURNEY WE MUST ALL MAKE

In 1989, Wangusa, a Mugisu from southern Bugisu, published a novel, *Upon this Mountain*, which tells the story of three Gisu boys from childhood to circumcision. One achieves the ordeal successfully, one fails and thereafter adopts the role of a transvestite and lastly, the narrator himself, having witnessed the humiliation of his friend, decides to take the schoolboy's still shameful option of having the operation done in hospital. Because of the insight this book gives, especially on early childhood experiences, I propose to quote it at some length in order to use it as the basis for future discussion. The novel opens with a vivid account of weaning, the first memory of the narrator, Mwambu, which is here reproduced in a slightly abridged form.

> Many, many millet granaries ago, he was mother's child, and she was the child's mother. And they sat in the shade on the verandah of the main house: mother with her legs stretched in front of her, to let the midday meal sink into her bones; and he fast asleep beside mother, with his head in mother's lap.[. . .]
> And he opened his eyes upon his mother: Mother's face, mother's arms, mother's lap. Tendermost mother as before. And he felt the itch inside him to suck at the breast. To clamber into her cosy, everysure lap and suck.
> 'Mother mine,' he said, rising and clambering. But as he reached out for the breast, he tripped over her legs and fell against her womb. And then came the rebuff.

'*Pthwoh*!' she spat into his face and pushed him away in visible anger. 'You a man!' His face went into a shocked, wide-mouthed, closed-eyed, noiseless contortion. . . . 'You such a grown-up! . . .'
Mother-bad-good-bad-good-why?
'. . . To go harassing me for my breast as if it was yours! And after you've just eaten so much food!'
And now the noiseless contortion broke into a shrill, loud and long cry of anguished bafflement.[. . .]
Everything reeled before him. Reeling millet granary. Reeling world. Trembling sky-line through the tear-drops. Mountain falling into the valleys and valleys falling onto mountain.
[. . .]His crying prompted even harsher retaliation and his mother beat him until . . . a very powerful voice saved him.
'Who is that beating Mwambu?' His father's voice! From the house. A strong and concerned voice.[. . .]
And instantly his toddling feet were fleeing from mother's presence to father's voice, through the instinctively remembered door. Before him was an outstretched arm. And now both arms. And then he found himself lifted by strong arms and placed on a strong soft bed. His father held him close to his breast and said:
'And now do not cry any more,
You are a man . . .
Do not cry, mother is bad . . .
I will beat her for you.' (Wangusa, 1989: 1–2)

Clearly, the value of this account does not rest on its literal accuracy as to whether weaning is always achieved in this sudden and harsh way. Rather, it gives vivid testimony to the psychic importance of the event; an insight into the effects of maternal rejection and also into the patterning of social relations and their cultural values. Of interest here is that the ambivalent feelings associated with weaning are, in this account, attributed solely to the mother. There is no paternal interdiction. Indeed, the male world is presented as the succouring one, the father aligning with his son against the – at that time – inexplicable cruelty of the mother. The novel records how he learnt that his rejection was due to his mother's pregnancy with his younger sister. Further, what is again striking about this account is that the rejection of the breast immediately qualifies the boy as a 'man', repeated by both the father and then by a cousin's wife, who offers him the sexual rewards of adulthood.

Some days later Mayaba, the newly-married wife of his cousin Kuloba, came into the courtyard, and threw him a challenge:
'How are you, husband of mine?' she asked. 'I hear that you're no

longer sucking mother's breast. You've done a very good thing. And it shows how very wise you are! You've seen that you're now a big man. And that's the truth. And on my part, I am myself now completely ready to be your wife. Tell me, aren't you happy? I'm happy myself. . . . Come, let's go to our house. Tonight you must share my bed with me. Come at once and let's go to our house. . . . Come let's go, I say. I am your wife. Your brother has gone on a journey today and I have no husband. You must come and keep his place in the bed warm. . . . Hey, are you running away? What are you afraid of? Poor me, what a husband!' (Wangusa, 1989: 3)

Reading this account it struck me that circumcision, replaying these same themes, might well draw some of its emotive power from them, and the tangle of emotions which is here presented as unresolved. Can we see in this weaning the symbolic castration that Lacan refers to? The child loses its mother but cannot yet assume the role of an adult and identify with his father or make the immediate transfer from non-genital to genital sexuality. He, in effect, enters a long period characterised by loss, where the mother is no longer 'mine' and clearly has to be shared with the father as well as with his other siblings. The process of autonomous self-development is now marked by a succession of movements away from the mother. From the 'mother mine' of infancy, the son continues to reside in the parental house but with a demoted status, sharing his mother with his father as well as other siblings. At 8 or 9 he makes a further move away when he moves out of the parental home. At this time he either builds himself a boy's house at the edge of his father's compound or goes to live with a friend.

Boys thus differentiate and achieve autonomy in a three-stage move: weaning, extrusion from the parental home and lastly circumcision. The time of his adolescence, when he lives apart from his parents, appears much as an interregnum in his relationship with them. During this time, he is largely freed from direct supervision and parental discipline, always somewhat erratic in Bugisu, is attenuated. Nevertheless, he has yet to gain a full social identity and is still regarded an adjunct to that of his parents. Thus, if ill-luck or illness strike him, this is seen as aimed not so much at himself as at his parents. Circumcision dramatically changes this state of affairs; like weaning it marks an abrupt change in his relationship to his parents. It is thus relevant to compare how his relationships with his mother and father are depicted in the ritual, and how they might relate to the weaning experience.

If we look firstly at the mother's role in the ritual, it is clear that she is presented as expediting her son's assumption of manhood and, in effect, as discussed earlier, 'rebirthing' him. Yet this is a rebirthing where the son himself is seen as the initiator of the process of separation. Circumcision thus effectively reverses the attitudes engendered by weaning as recorded by Wangusa. The mother now is presented in a totally positive light and the separation which marks his final exit from the maternal home is presented as a matter of *his choice*, albeit facilitated by his mother.

There are interesting and important contrasts with the father's role. Again, ideally, the father is presented as nurturant, ensuring his son's safe and successful circumcision by choosing the ritual elder (often himself), the circumcisor and making sure that no ill-will remains in the family which could threaten the boy's welfare. However, he remains on the side lines, responsible for practical arrangements but not implicated in the actual process whereby his son achieves his manhood. In this, he is rather like the bride's mother in an English wedding and again, like her, he is given no direct role in the ritual itself. Indeed, it is not even important that he be present as long as he has given his permission for it to go ahead, for circumcisions can be performed also at the house of any senior relative, matrilateral as well as patrilineal. But, in any event, the father's role is tinged with ambiguity for the very powers he is entrusted with to ensure his son's well-being are subject to abuse. Thus, when a boy fails in the ordeal, fails to show the requisite courage or fails in afterlife and does not manage to maintain a marriage, then directly or indirectly the father may be deemed at fault. No such blame attaches to the mother whose fortitude is always linked in a positive way to that of her son. The same applies also to the sisters who identify strongly with their brothers as they accompany them on the three days leading to circumcision.

A question which may be addressed here is why is the mother idealised? Given the account of weaning, with its horrifying images of alienation and loss of security, a loss which the novel implies is never repaired, why do we not find images of evil female power? We may here refer to the work of Klein who stresses the conflicting attitude of the child to the breast as both the source of libidinal satisfaction and the primary source of frustration. Frustration she held to be inevitable because of the nature of infantile narcissism and omnipotence. The image of the 'bad breast' and bad mother then becomes the 'prototype of all persecuting and frightening objects' (Klein, 1989: 66), a product of the child's aggressive phantasies, which is later carried over to the penis. For Klein, the transfer to genital sexuality is never total and the attitude taken to the breast underwrites the possibility of successful adaptation to mature sexual identity, of a positive attitude to the penis. In Wangusa's account of weaning, the substitution of the penis for the nipple is clearly depicted, as is the ambivalence to the mother. Perhaps, we may also see in the symbolism of the knife which 'eats' the boy's penis at circumcision an indication of oral/sadistic phantasy, a product of the guilt inspired in the child who, through the introjection of threatening parental images, turns his own aggressive phantasies against himself. Circumcision then is not necessarily solely a representation of 'castration' inflicted by fathers but equally, and perhaps more, a representation of the phantasies inspired by maternal rejection.

Whether or not such an interpretation, resting on the intangibility of infantile sexual phantasy, is valid, we can still unite Klein and Lacan with Wangusa and see weaning as the first encounter of the child with the reality principle. Circumcision might then be seen as the test of whether the individual has faced this crisis successfully. The pain of the rejection at weaning is matched by the physical pain borne at circumcision and the necessity for the individual to prove he can cope with the hardships and deprivations of life.

To return to the question as to why the representation of hostility to the mother might be subdued we need again to refer to the structural situation which creates a very real dependence of men upon women. The Gisu inherit through the house-property complex; that is, a man has a right only to those fields farmed by his own mother, a prerogative which is especially important in a polygamous household. Mothers are thus crucial intermediaries in a man's struggle to gain his inheritance from his father. Thus, the rival claims of son and father to the loyalty and affection of the mother continue after circumcision; both must vie for her primary loyalty. The same situation applies to sisters and wives. A man's chances of marrying a wife depend in great measure on having a younger sister or sisters, as he has a priority claim on their bridewealth. Without such sisters his chances of an early marriage, essential to the establishment of a full adult identity, are prejudiced. Without a wife he cannot maintain an independent household successfully or have children to establish his status and his line of descent. Yet, to a large extent, the Gisu give women the same freedoms as accord to men and this results in a fairly high divorce rate, especially in the early years. Successful marriages thus depend on negotiation, particularly in the most problematic areas which relate to the disposal of the products of their joint labour. Where marriage breaks down it is invariably held to be the husband's fault and here it is significant that, unlike the surrounding peoples, the Gisu do not consider that men have an automatic or 'natural' right to beat their wives. Indeed, wife beating is subject to general condemnation and provides grounds for a wife to sue her husband in court or to divorce him.

Men's relationships with women are thus coloured by insecurity. Women are the essential helpmates but a man must vie with his father over the loyalty of his mother and with other men to retain the loyalty of his wife. Can we see in this the source of the repression of hostility to the mother at *imbalu*? Put in a psychodynamic context, we could say (though, as an anthropologist, no more than tentatively) that the idealisation of the mother is a defensive projection, consequent on the first insoluble dilemma posed to the infant who, despite his mother's inexplicable (and to the child, capricious) rejection, must continue to rely and depend upon her. Circumcision, as the final act of individuation, changes some of the terms present during weaning but not all. The boy is now presented as choosing emancipation and is 'freed', yet, in actuality, his dependence on his parents continues after circumcision. Can we see this ambiguity as being resolved, at least in part, by canalising hostile feelings towards the father? This might be one of the paradoxical implications of the rite: the boy 'saves' the mother at least partially for himself but the consequences are that he projects all his aggression onto his father and the male world which now includes himself. Autonomous manhood can be won only by means of a sacrifice but it is a sacrifice in which a man takes on responsibility for the hostility in the world.

GENDER RELATIONS

Given the hostility which is seen to dominate the world of men in contrast to the world of women, this section looks further at the way in which gender relationships are depicted at *imbalu*. One of the more unusual features of *imbalu* is the way in which it valorises the male gender and masculine heroism but in such a way as to draw the sexes together rather than radically to oppose them. The image of complementarity is sustained. If women are weaker than men it is because they do not face the knife but this does not detract from their identification with the ritual. For example, the main myth associated with circumcision relates how the practice originated in a marriage with a woman from a neighbouring people who also circumcise women. When this woman began circumcising her daughters, the men saw that it made them 'too strong' and so started circumcising themselves instead. But, if men thus checked the physical power of women, they did not take away the power altogether, for *imbalu* is still held to be transmitted through women as well as through men, and the myth relates how the practice spread throughout the country as a result of intermarriage.

Nevertheless, the linking of circumcision with male violence and with sexuality through the fermentation metaphor raises the question of how far, in other respects, violence is linked to sex. This theme is undoubtedly present in Bugisu, as elsewhere, but is not greatly elaborated. The equation of circumcision with virility and warriorhood is given in a common metaphor used in Kenya, that of the penis as the 'sharpened spear', trimmed for use against both other men and, of course, women. I never heard this used in Bugisu and, indeed, it could well be that the Gisu lie at the opposite extreme to some of the cultures of Kenya with their explicit gender antagonism, with all sex seen as a form of rape (see LeVine, 1959). Rather, Gisu circumcision rituals seem to proclaim a separation here by putting the emphasis on the military rather than the sexual role of men. The complementarity of the sexes and the necessity of their co-operation remains the keynote.

Circumcision does, however, provide a symbolic resource for commenting upon the relative powers of the sexes. It creates, as does any complex social practice, a number of different dimensions, whose messages can be read in contrasting directions. The rites thus provide an image not only for gender asymmetry but also for gender symmetry, pulling the sexes together in so doing. For example, if one looks at the castrating aspects in the dimension of pain endured, then the Gisu directly relate circumcision to childbirth. Boys are exhorted to 'stand like a woman giving birth' and the whole process, as I have outlined, puts circumcision on a par with procreation. Both men and women have experience of pain but their emotional responses to it are different. Women retain their compassion and their ability to identify with others; men are hardened by the experience and lose their compassion. In so doing, men achieve power over women. However, if one looks at circumcision in terms of blood letting, as Bettelheim (1954) has argued, then women come out as naturally superior for, whereas it is said that men bleed only once, women are said to bleed twice. The bleeding identified here is the blood of menstruation and the blood of parturition. With respect to fertility women thus have the edge. But, again, in terms of the blood of 'spoiling', both sexes come out as equivalent; both must be 'spoilt' so they can engage in a successful and fertile adult life.

These themes played out in the ritual context give rise to its characteristic ambiguities and paradoxes. The primary one in this context is that in making a boy a man it also makes a boy *more* like a woman; not only is he identified with women 'helpers' but in the course of the ritual, he must bleed, be passive and be spoilt. Indeed, at the time of the operation the boy is essentially androgynous, combining both male and female positions, active and passive, male and castrated male. He must prove his maturity in the same way as women by being spoilt by men; the operation condensing into one symbol all the aspects of feminine maturity: bleeding, defloration, gestation and birth. If he becomes a man and not a woman it is because of what women are deemed to lack in this process – aggressivity. But he does not by so doing extend male mastery into the area of reproduction. The Gisu boy is made to put himself in the position of women; he does not arrogate their powers. The 'bisexuality' of the symbolism points in a rather different direction, one which again takes us back to the Freudian postulate as to the original identification of child with the mother and the play of both feminine and masculine identifications in the personality structures of both men and women.

If we regard circumcision as a maturation experience, a *test* of adulthood, then can we also read its symbolism as providing the materials for individual adjustment? One possibility suggested by the psychoanalyst Florence Bégoin-Guignard is that it might provide the opportunity for the equivalent of a transference experience.[7] Thus, we might see its symbols as allowing for the displacement of conflicts and, as in the analytic encounter, the possibility for a reworking of them in new terms. The ritual might then truly be seen to provide the occasion for personal growth: an opportunity which individuals would respond to and use differently. The promise of such an approach comes from the fact that we could then give adequate weight to both the individual and the cultural in our analyses of the rite and its effects. The fuller elaboration of such an approach is beyond the scope of this paper, but its attraction lies in its potential to develop much further the themes which are present in the ritual and the way in which these are actually handled by Gisu individuals, for example, those of sexuality and gender identity, of pain, loss and suffering, of the fusion between aggression and sexuality, of the play between destruction and creation, of choice versus constraint and of independence versus submission.

At this point, we may return to the Oedipal dilemma and ask if the 'spoiling' of people could be taken in a wider metaphoric way? This is the theme of the last section.

EVERY MAN A HERO

Freud's writings on culture remained important to him throughout his life and he never abandoned the account of the origins of religion that he had formulated in *Totem and Taboo*. Thus, he held that religion owed its origin and obsessional character to the return or unconscious memory of an act of parricide. 'Men have always known . . . that once upon a time they had a primaeval father and killed him' (1951: 161). To expurgate the deed, appease the dead father and to allay the sense of guilt born with it, the parricidal sons began to honour the totem as the substitute for the father and renounced the fruits of their act by resigning their claim to the women of the group. Thus the primary rules of social life – the taboos on in-group murder and incest – were born. The taboos represent both the desired and the forbidden and answer to the dilemma in all of us of instinct versus the demands of social living. According to this account, circumcision is an act of sacrifice, signifying submission to the father's will, to the incest taboo, and thus to culture.

The reading of circumcision as an act of repressive socialisation is plausible in many cultural contexts, especially in those based on patriarchal geronto-cracies, but does not seem to be particularly applicable to the Gisu because of the lack of a strong system of paternal authority. In turn, this raises more general problems about the application of Freudian theory with its stress on the role of the father and the paternal imaging of cultural legitimacy. This is the case whether one takes the orthodox line or, alternatively, regards the account as 'myth', that is an allegorical statement about the existential necessities for the achievement of personal autonomy and culture. Even if, after Lacan, we take it that it is the *idea* of paternal power which is important, this problem still holds, for he, no less than Freud, sees the assumption of individuality, of personhood, to lie in the Oedipal dynamic. Lemaire (1977) offers the following summary of Lacan's views:

> The Oedipus is the drama of a being who must become a subject and who can only do so by internalizing the social rules, by entering on an equal footing into the register of the symbolic, of Culture and of language; it is the drama of a future subject who must resolve the problem of the difference between the sexes, of the assumption of his or her own sex and of his or her unconscious drives by means of a development which presupposes the transition from natural man to man of culture. (Lemaire, 1977: 91–2)

Oedipal conflict must happen for the individual to realise his humanity. If this is so, then circumcision should by these accounts at least provide some representation of it. And, at this point, I should say that it is possible to find this theme in the ritual. We can indeed interpret the rite as initiated by a symbolic killing of the father which is followed by the identification of mother and son in sexual union. This is finally countered by the offer of a wife and reinforced by a symbolic castration as the boy faces the knife.

The first ritual act of the circumcision ritual is, as has been mentioned earlier, the threshing of the millet which marks the boy's intent. Imme-diately following this, the boy and his party go into one of the father's banana plantations where the boy knocks down a bunch of bananas by smashing the stem of the tree with his bare hands. This act requires considerable strength and is met with shouts of approval. The bananas are then roasted and eaten together with a sacrificial chicken. This act is never interpreted and banana symbolism is not otherwise used in the ritual. However, the destruction of the main stem may be interpreted as a sym-bolic marker of the end of one life and the beginning of a new, represented in the basal shoots growing to replace the old (and now destroyed) stem. As such it represents the divide at which the boy finds himself, but it may also be read for messages about the father and son relationship. Indeed, the death of the old and its replacement by the new generation could hardly be more vividly depicted and, if we follow this line of reasoning, then the smashing of the stem becomes an act of symbolic parricide.

Following this, and throughout the ritual process, mother and son become increasingly identified through the making of the circumcision beer, an act usually performed by husband and wife. Further, the image of the boy pouring water on the prepared millet could be read as an image of intercourse. For this task he must take a traditional round clay pot and fetch water from a stream or spring, carrying it back on his head without the use of a headrest. This water he then pours onto the prepared beer millet held in a much larger clay pot, immediately changing it from inert matter to a bubbling mixture. Again it is possible to read this as a representation of the boy's sexuality, with the water providing an image of semen and masculinity, while the millet represents the receptive powers of femininity. The Gisu do link men to rain and to water and women to the earth. To continue, this is followed by the boy being smeared with yeast by a senior agnate (never by his own father) together with his sisters, while the yeast is added by his mother to the brew. As has been said, this act can be taken as signifying gestation. Lastly, there is the operation itself, a 'birth' on the part of the mother, and a simultaneous death and rebirth for the son. Not implausibly, following this line of exposition, it may also be read as an act of punishment inflicted by the collectivity of Gisu men on the boy for his incestuous desires.

The crucial problem with this line of interpretation is that the Gisu do not offer any commentary along these lines. To make this interpretation then we have to accept the fact of repression. However, there are evident problems for the anthropologist here because of the difference between his or her task and material and that used by the psychoanalyst. In therapeutic work, as in ritual, the dynamic adduced is that of cathartic abreaction. In order for this to be effective psychologically, the process demands an element of at least subliminal recognition, the conflict represented, as Devereux (1961) puts it, 'in a form acceptable to the ego'. It is this thesis which has frequently aroused the most anthropological hostility because of its supposed identification of cultural rituals with neurotic individual ones. Nor do we as anthropologists have access to material as to subliminal recognition. Unlike psychoanalysts, for whom interpretative support is provided in the dynamics of the analytic encounter and particularly in the fact of transference, anthropologists are more heavily reliant on the hypothetical surmise. This, it seems to me, remains an insoluble problem for this form of interpretation.

Further, even if we accept the Oedipal reading, we have some problems of interpretation. For example, in the most usual case, the boy stands *imbalu* facing his father. Do we read this as an act of submission or an act of insubordination, the boy standing against his father and outfacing him? Or does it partake of both attitudes? Again, the problem of interpretation here, as is the problem throughout when dealing with the Gisu data, relates to the weak imaging of paternal power. If it were strong, there would be less hesitation about giving a straightforward Oedipal reading and identifying the father with authority and with tradition. But, in the Gisu case, there is a stronger argument that it is the boy and not the father who is taken to embody tradition. His desire to take *imbalu* is seen as a direct inspiration and an embodiment of ancestral power. Thus, he is regarded as having been 'caught' by the ancestral power of circumcision: simultaneously making manifest and submitting to the potentialities of his birth and identity. And again, the ancestral power of circumcision, like all the ancestral powers, is not identified with patriarchal authority. These powers are not fully personified but represent the continuity of ancestry, associated in a general way with the unremembered spirits of the dead, both maternal and paternal. They are not wished down by living agency but 'catch' those within their orbit.

At this point, one may take a sideways look at the process. In *Moses and Monotheism*, Freud discusses the image of the hero and its role in the creation of the idea of a high god and the particular forms of conscience recognised in both Judaism and in Christianity. Yet, his depiction of the hero or great man is also apposite here for his characterisation is strongly reminiscent of qualities all Gisu men claim for themselves. To quote from just one passage, Freud writes of the 'decisiveness of thought, the strength of will, the forcefulness of his deeds' and of 'the self-reliance and independence of the great man: his conviction of doing the right thing, which must pass into ruthlessness' (1951: 174). For Freud these characterisations belong to the picture of the archetypal father but this is not necessary. Indeed, as he mentions in another passage, 'A hero is a man who stands up manfully against his own father and in the end victoriously overcomes him' (Freud, 1951: 18).

Gisu circumcision is a dramatic act of individuation: a boy makes himself a man. He sets himself up against his father and is circumcised standing opposite to him. In so doing he proves identity and parity with his father but, equally, he takes on the burden of culture and commits himself bodily to it. Thus, it also presents itself as a dramatic act of conversion, attendant on the incorporation of what Fortes once called 'wild youth' into the main body of society. This theme is present in the circumcision regalia, whose sole purpose is said to make the boy look wild, and in other imagery, such as referring to the penis at this time as '*isolo*', the wild animal. From being outside the law, the boy is being made to submit to it, albeit in an act represented as being of his own volition.

May we here speculate that egalitarian cultures may have a particular need for heroes which make each individual the bearer not only of culture, but of a culture that is depicted as harsh and onerous? This is reminiscent of Stanner's (1963) view that Australian Aboriginal religion expresses a deep concern with a paradox central to the meaning of life, which is that the 'good life' depends upon people being willing to suffer injury. Hiatt (1975), in commenting upon this and drawing upon the work of Roheim, goes further and argues that Australian totemism and its ritual represent 'protoanalytical insights' and display significant understanding of the problems of growing up and the conditions of the unconscious. I would not want to press this claim for the Gisu but I do think it is possible to see Gisu circumcision, as outlined in the previous section, as a test for the autonomy and self-responsibility attendant upon adulthood which rests upon the individual's ability to have overcome his infantile conflicts and achieved adequate separation from the mother; thus, to have come to terms with reality and the loss and pain this involves. Almost the worst act a boy can commit during the actual operation is to call out for his mother or father. This is seen to be as polluting as falling to the ground and likewise regarded as an act of destruction, both of himself and of his family.

The father's words in Wangusa's story, 'And now do not cry any more. You are a man', are apposite here and, in effect, summarise the whole process. The importance of the individual nature of the test is apparent in the fear of failure which runs through it. The image and threat of failure are never allowed to go away during the long build-up to the operation. While this can be seen, on the one hand, as a fairly direct process of 'battle-proofing' (see Heald, 1986), the other side of this is to exaggerate the element of the 'test' and to highlight failure. Other peoples in Kenya, who equally insist on circumcision as a test of fortitude, do not elaborate upon the preparatory period to the same extent. Indeed, it is common for children to leave for the ceremonial sites with little or no ritual preparation and the main celebrations then follow the operation. Yet, these children are just as stoic as the Gisu and possibly even more so. For example, among the Kuria of south-west Kenya, the shamefulness of failure is considered so great that it is thought of as almost an impossibility. By contrast, a relatively large number of Gisu boys do fail. I have estimated that two or three out of ten do not stand the ordeal with the required degree of fortitude and even more try to evade it or put it off for so long that they risk being cut by force. The test of the mettle of the individual is thus certainly a very real one.

This leads me to a more general point. In previous publications, I have broached the problem of how social order is maintained in systems such as that of the Gisu where the authority principle is weak. I have argued that the onus is then put on self-control. Where there are no coercive authorities to enforce the law the individual is seen as the bearer of restriction much more strongly than in authoritarian cultures. The restrictions on individual freedom are imaged in the absoluteness of taboo tied to kinship and ancestry. Nevertheless, even here, morality is governed by pragmatics rather than by precept alone. The boundaries of custom, when determined through ancestral power, are changeable and each individual must, in a sense, test them out for him or herself. This makes the regulations of kinship important not only for what they explicitly prohibit but for how they should be read as general messages about the relationship of self to others. As I have argued (Heald, 1989, 1990), these messages relate to the importance of self-denial and the necessity to exercise restraint in both sexuality and aggression.

The messages of circumcision are more ambiguous because of the power of violence which it is seen to entail. But, in undergoing *imbalu*, the boy clearly is making an unconditional statement of his place in the line of tradition and recognising its validity. In so doing, he recognises its pain and its enduring power in the marks which will be permanently inscribed on his body and in the forceful power which is now his. The 'spoiling' image is indeed apt. Circumcision, as is repeatedly said, is a bitter thing. In becoming a man, he takes on responsibility for self and, in so doing, he also takes on responsibility for the harshness of the world, a responsibility he shares with all men. To that extent every man must be a hero.

NOTES

1 I am indebted to Reg Hook for helping to clarify a number of issues in this paper in the stimulating discussions we had in Canberra in 1991, and to Florence Bégoin-Guignard and Vincent Crapanzano for their perceptive comments on this paper during and after the Paris colloquium.
2 While the phylogenetic implications of Freud's *Totem and Taboo* have usually been dropped in favour of the ontogenetic, this line of argument, though with variations as to stress, is to be found in the earlier work of Roheim (e.g. 1934), Whiting, Kluckhohn and Anthony (1958) and more recently in Spiro (1982) and Ottenberg (1988).
3 See especially, Fortes, 1966, 1977, and Turner, 1967.
4 Though, at the same time, it is possible to see it as an occasion when men are able to display their complementary Oedipal aggression (see Spiro, 1982) in both their taunts and their identification with individual candidates.
5 This prohibition is given its greatest expression in the avoidance of relationships of a man with his mother-in-law and daughter-in-law. These relationships, as I have described, serve as prototypes for all forbidden sexual relationships (Heald, 1990).
6 Their area of competition is that of the 'penis' (*ihando*), the word used of heritable property. By contrast the property exchanges that accompany marriage are referred to as '*buxwe*', a term which is also used of sexual shame.
7 Private communication.

208   *Working models*

BIBLIOGRAPHY

Bettelheim, B. (1954) *Symbolic Wounds*. Glencoe, Ill.: The Free Press.
Cohen, P. (1980) 'Psychoanalysis and cultural symbolization', in M. L. Foster and S. H. Brandes (eds) *Symbol as Sense*. London: Academic Press.
Devereux, G. (1961) 'Art and mythology: a general theory', in B. Kaplan (ed.) *Studying Personality Cross-Culturally*. Illinois: Row, Peterson.
Fortes, M. (1966) 'Totem and taboo', *Proceedings of the Royal Anthropological Institute* 5–22.
―― (1977) 'Custom and conscience in anthropological perspective', *International Review of Psycho-Analysis* 4: 127–54.
Freud, S. (1950 [1912–13]) *Totem and Taboo*. London: Routledge & Kegan Paul.
―― (1951 [1933–4]) *Moses and Monotheism*. London: The Hogarth Press.
Heald, S. S. (1982) 'The making of men: the relevance of vernacular psychology to the interpretation of a Gisu ritual', *Africa* 52: 15–36.
―― (1986) 'The ritual use of violence: circumcision among the Gisu of Uganda', in D. Riches (ed.) *The Anthropology of Violence*. Oxford: Blackwell.
―― (1989) *Controlling Anger: The Sociology of Gisu Violence*. Manchester and New York: Manchester University Press/St Martin's Press.
―― (1990) 'Joking and avoidance, hostility and incest: an essay on Gisu moral categories', *Man* ns 25: 377–92.
Hiatt, L. R. (1975) Introduction to L. R. Hiatt (ed.) *Australian Aboriginal Mythology*. Canberra: Australian Institute for Aboriginal Studies.
Klein, M. (1989 [1945]) 'The Oedipus complex in the light of early anxieties', reprinted in R. Britton *et al.* (eds) *The Oedipus Complex Today*. London: Karnac.
Lacan, J. (1977) *Ecrits: A Selection*, trans. A. Sheridan. London: Tavistock.
La Fontaine, J. (1967) 'Parricide in Bugisu: a study in intergenerational conflict', *Man* ns 2: 249–59.
Leach, E. (1958) 'Magical hair', *Journal of the Royal Anthropological Institute* 77: 147–64.
Lemaire, A. (1977) *Jacques Lacan*. London: Routledge & Kegan Paul.
LeVine, R. A. (1959) 'Gusii sex offences', *American Anthropologist* 61: 965–90.
Ottenberg, S. (1988) 'Oedipus, gender and social solidarity: a case study of male childhood and initiation', *Ethos* 16: 326–52.
Reik, T. (1931) *Ritual*. London: The Hogarth Press.
Ricoeur, P. (1979) 'Psychoanalysis and the movement of contemporary culture', in P. Rabinow and W. M. Sullivan (eds) *Interpretive Social Science: A Reader*. Berkeley: University of California Press.
―― (1981) 'The question of proof in Freud's psychoanalytical writings', in J. B. Thompson (ed.) *Paul Ricoeur: Hermeneutics and the Human Sciences*. Cambridge: Cambridge University Press.
Roheim, G. (1934) *The Riddle of the Sphinx or Human Origins*. London: The Hogarth Press.
Spiro, M. E. (1982) *Oedipus in the Trobriands*. London and Chicago: University of Chicago Press.
Stanner, W. E. H. (1963) *On Aboriginal Religion*. Oceania Monograph 11. Sydney: University of Sydney.
Stephens, W. N. (and D'Andrade) (1962) *The Oedipus Complex*. New York: Free Press of Glencoe.

Turner, V. W. (1967) 'Symbols in Ndembu ritual', in *Forest of Symbols*. Ithaca, NY: Cornell University Press, pp. 19–47.
Wangusa, T. (1989) *Upon This Mountain*. London: Heinemann.
Whiting, J. W., Kluckhohn, R. and Anthony, A. (1958) 'The function of male initiation ceremonies at puberty', in E. Maccoby, W. Newcomb and R. Hartley (eds) *Readings in Social Psychology*. New York: Holt, Rinehart & Winston.

13 Symbolic homosexuality and cultural theory

The unconscious meaning of sister exchange among the Gimi of Highland New Guinea

Gillian Gillison

In an article first published in France in 1965, Devereux complained that the circulation of women in marriage – the phenomenon Lévi-Strauss described as generating *The Elementary Structures of Kinship* – hardly explained the origin of kinship in human society. To understand matrimonial exchanges and the 'infrastructure of kinship systems', Devereux said, it was necessary to pass from purely sociological discourse into the realm of psychoanalysis. The moment 'certain general psychological and cultural facts' are combined, he argued, the exchange of women in marriage expresses not merely the law of talion or a system of *prestations mutuelles* (Mauss, 1967), but 'an obsessional tendency toward *"bilanisme"* . . . a compulsive quest for symmetry' that is the hallmark of latent male homosexuality (Devereux, 1978: 204). It is always men who exchange women in marriage – never the converse – according to Devereux because men's homosexual fantasies lie at the heart of kinship systems. 'Kinship is not rooted in heterosexual but in homosexual drives', he said (ibid.: 209). The institution of marriage repels 'the threatening specter of latent homosexuality' by allowing men to achieve their goal in symbolic form, disguising homosexuality 'as a heterosexual act'. 'Marriage is sacred, that is: dangerous, precisely because it permits what is forbidden; it consecrates a sacrilege' (ibid.: 211).

Devereux realised that his 'addendum' to Lévi-Strauss' theory, which turned the deep structure of kinship into an avoidance – and thus a covert expression – of male homosexuality, was a 'singular' idea, and he states at the beginning and end of his article that he hesitated for years to publish it (ibid.: 180, 212). But he sounds disingenuous, or anxious to please his mentor, when he insists that his 'analysis is perfectly compatible with Lévi-Strauss' structural analysis' and that 'those who might try to oppose his theory of kinship and mine, or inversely, will labor in vain' (1978: 211–12). Certainly, Lévi-Strauss' demonstration that marriage regulations 'do not concern the relationship between men and women but between the men themselves' and that 'women are simply their objects' is consistent, in the strict sense, with Devereux' premise that those regulations have an unconsciously homosexual motive. But any psychoanalytic interpretation of kinship is bound to conflict with Lévi-Strauss' analysis because it is based upon a wholly different concept of the unconscious: one that injects purpose, intentionality, affect, etc., into 'deep structures' that Lévi-Strauss insists are neutral and content-free. From a psychoanalytic perspective, unconscious sexual fantasies have a determining role in the organisation of social institutions like kinship and marriage. Unlike Devereux, and in company with most anthropologists, Lévi-Strauss vehemently rejects the relevance of psychoanalysis to his theories, claiming that the study of individuals, or the individual psyche, can shed no light upon the inner workings of social systems (e.g., 1977, 1988).

Classic social anthropology, founded in the work of Durkheim, takes as its object of study the whole social organism, an entity composed not of individuals but of institutions like kinship, language and religion, 'social facts' that are external to individuals and therefore 'objective' and 'obligatory' (Durkheim, 1966). While it is true that there could be no social life without the psychical functions of individuals, the old argument runs, social processes are intrinsically different from the phenomena of individual psychology. They 'transcend [individual] functions . . . and, if not independent of mind, have an existence of their own outside individual minds' (Evans-Pritchard, 1965: 55). Traditional anthropology is set against a psychology derived from Freud or, indeed, against any anthropology that views society as a collection of individuals, its institutions the reflection of problems, both fantasied and real, that individuals share (e.g., Douglas, 1970: 137–65).

But my purpose here is not to examine the theoretical impasse between psychoanalysis and anthropology or between the work of Devereux and of Lévi-Strauss. It is rather to provide data from my own fieldwork among the Gimi of Highland Papua New Guinea which (despite the fact that I had no knowledge of Devereux until some fifteen years after my first contact with the Gimi) amply confirm Devereux's thesis about the homosexual meaning of marriage and thus argue for the relevance of psychoanalysis to the understanding of social rules and 'facts'.[1] If the human psyche includes an unconscious, and if the unconscious works in the way Freud described, then the findings of psychoanalysis bear upon every kind of human activity. The Durkheimian concept of an over-arching, superorganic and fundamentally other level of reality, one that is immortal, objective, etc., because external to the individual, or the individual mind, is as resistant to demonstration, and certainly more mystical, than Freud's idea of the unconscious. But, unlike the unconscious, the notion of the superorganic tends to create a harmonious view of human social life, one in which political and religious institutions are mechanically reproduced. By positing an autonomous, self-perpetuating social realm, and insisting that it alone constitutes the true and proper field of enquiry, anthropologists created the pretext to dismiss – under the misnomer 'individual' – the sexual content of human fantasy and behaviour, labelling as 'private' or 'psychological' the collective attitudes and myths which often lie at the heart of social conflict (e.g., Leach, 1967).

Devereux begins his reinterpretation of Lévi-Strauss' theory about the origin of kinship with the Oedipus complex because 'the Oedipus complex is inseparable from the notion of kinship' (Devereux, 1978: 180–1). Although the Oedipus complex is 'first and foremost a psychosocial phenomenon', Devereux says, it has a 'physiological dimension': whereas female animals experience phases of rutting and maternity, a woman may be simultaneously sexual and maternal. 'A pregnant or lactating woman can continue to be wife or lover, while a bitch or a cow, in the same state, is entirely mother . . . the sexualization of maternity is at the root of the Oedipus complex' (ibid.: 182–3). Many peoples devise taboos and restrictions to desynchronise the two phases of female sexuality. 'Very many tribes forbid sexual relations during pregnancy and lactation: the woman must be wife or mother, but never both simultaneously' (ibid.: 183).

Juxtaposing clinical, ethnographic and classical material, Devereux sets up a link between the coincidence of women's sexual and reproductive functions and men's Oedipal fantasies, specifically the tendency to identify wife with mother. A man tends to imagine his every sex partner as also a mother, as one who *already* has a husband, an attitude that turns every sexual encounter into a kind of threesome: 'to mount a woman is to mount her spouse, her father and her brother'. The inclusion of a woman's 'husband' or 'husbands' – even if she is unmarried and a virgin, her 'husbands' being nothing other than spectres of her own incestuous wishes – causes injury to them. 'The fact of being mounted soils the honor of the *woman*, but *even more* and perhaps *primarily*, that of the men of her family' (ibid.: 192). As Devereux notes, 'a normal woman does not feel humiliated when she makes love . . . it is not the woman's humiliation through coitus which explains the shame of her kinsmen; on the contrary, it is the latter which explains the former' (ibid.: 195).

This humiliation or injury to the men of a woman's family, though committed on the level of fantasy, has to be compensated for in reality, through the reciprocal organisation of marriage, because '[s]ociety cannot afford the luxury of ignoring so violent an internal conflict' (ibid.: 196). Exchanges of women, brideprice, brideservice, etc., are thus designed to repair – in a mutual and bilateral way – damages one man inflicts upon another by the fact of possessing, or intending to possess, his sister or daughter. In the same way, marriage rites themselves are contrived 'to disguise the outrage suffered by the "victim of theft" and to underplay the triumph of the "thief" (ibid.). The idea that one man harms another or steals something vital from him in the very act of copulating with the other's sister or daughter is inseparable, according to Devereux, from the notion that, for a man, heterosexual union always implicates a 'second man' – one who is already there, ensconced inside the woman – and who thus participates in the penetration or 'receives the penis' in the same moment as the woman. Sex with a woman combines in a man 'the hostile fantasy of causing injuries to her first "owner" (father, brother, husband) on the one hand and a homosexual fantasy of coitus with the "owner" on the other hand' (ibid.: 208).

According to Devereux, the circulation of women in marriage, and the kinship systems which Lévi-Strauss rests upon it, are attempts to make restitution for losses men inflict upon each other in the Oedipal fantasies that accompany their heterosexual relations, fantasies of a man's penetrating a woman's invisible prior husband or father. The institutions of marriage and kinship repel 'the threatening specter of latent homosexuality' between men who stand in a symbolic relation of father and son by realising the fantasy in a disguised and socially productive form. The unconscious meaning of marriage is of fruitful homosexual alliance, one that incorporates, in a reciprocal and bilateral way, fantasies of 'homosexual triumph over the father [that] is a *sine qua non* stage in the resolution, or sublimation, of the boy's Oedipus complex' (ibid.: 190).

Whatever its validity as a universal postulate, Devereux's set of associations seems to fit the Gimi case and to account for a wealth of detail in marriage ritual. Unlike men in some New Guinea societies (e.g., Williams, 1969 [1936]; Kelly, 1976; Schiefflin, 1976; Herdt, 1981; etc.), Gimi men do not practise ritual homosexuality and deny that they engage in homosexual acts. Gajdusek reports no overt homosexuality among Gimi men (diary entry); and over a period of nearly twenty years, during trips into the forest to photograph Birds of Paradise, David Gillison observed 'no sign or hint' of homosexual conduct or conversation. When, prodded by me, he put the question directly, men replied that they were not dogs, and did not 'act like dogs – nor like men in the Sepik!' Although one man alluded to the time when 'a Big Man is sweet on a young boy', he refused afterwards to elaborate (see note 1). Whatever the 'facts' about Gimi men's sexual conduct, they have little direct bearing upon the connection I draw between fantasy and social organisation. Taking my cue from Devereux, I attempt to link a *symbolic* homosexuality, implicit in Gimi myths and rites, not with the incidence of such behaviour in real life, but with the driving logic of marriage and exchange.

Two prominent themes of Gimi ritual are relevant to Devereux's argument. The first is a pervasive attempt to separate or 'desynchronise' women's reproductive and sexual functions, not only through elaborate pre-partum and post-partum taboos but also through marriage and the accompanying exchange of sacred bamboo flutes as secret icons of the brides.

THE SECRET OF THE FLUTES ACCORDING TO MEN

Gimi flutes are called 'birds' and men keep them in the rafters of their club houses, forbidding women and children to see them on pain of death (cf. Read, 1952, 1965; Salisbury, 1965; Langness, 1974; Herdt, 1981; etc.). In the late 1950s and early 1960s, missionaries arrived in Gimi territory just ahead of or behind the Australian patrols. Often they entered the men's houses, carried out the flutes, showed them to assembled women and children, burned them and then baptised the whole village. They also forbade the construction of men's houses and insisted that the new Christians live together in nuclear families. But, by 1973, the year of my first fieldwork, Gimi men were beginning to rebuild the men's houses, to make flutes and to initiate their adolescent sons.

Traditionally, women are married during the initiation of their younger brothers in a series of sister exchanges, and, though forbidden to see the flutes, transport them to their husbands 'unknowingly' on the day of their marriages. The fathers of the brides disguise the instruments as containers of salt or cooked meat and conceal them inside the brides' net bags. Each flute, or pair of flutes, is an icon of the bride who carries it on her back: markings her father etched around the blowing hole are of the same design as the 'beard' he recently had tattooed around her mouth. The blowing hole of a flute is a 'vagina', men reveal; the hollow chamber is a 'womb'; and the emerging sounds are 'cries' of a newborn child. A man's breath or 'wind' is his 'penis', the men say, and the movement of wind – the player's inhaling and blowing into the 'mouth' of the instrument – is an explicit metaphor for the back and forth movement of coitus. The flutes a man gives to his son-in-law consist not only of the instruments themselves, lengths of bamboo that will some day rot and have to be remade, but also of the right to play his own named 'cry', a distinctive combination of sounds and contrapuntal rhythms.

In the gift of his flute and flute 'cry', a man gives away both his daughter and the right to 'play' her his way. A man's 'blowing into a flute', men allow, 'is like going into a woman'.

A man's wind is his penis. . . . We saw woman's vagina and made a hole in the bamboo and added marks like pubic hair. Blowing into the mouth [of the flute with one's hand covering the end] is like penetration and [releasing the hand and] letting out the sound is like pushing the child out of the mother's vagina. That's why [demonstrating on an imaginary instrument] the blowing hole is small and the crying hole is big: one is the vagina for having sex and the other is the vagina for bearing the child.

Symbolised as flute playing, the male procreative role is to 'blow in' and 'blow out' a child. And men speak of actual conception and parturition in similar terms, describing the 'work' of a man in installing the child and inducing the birth. A man 'places the child' in a woman's belly through repeated acts of intercourse and, after a period of abstinence that lasts for nearly the whole of the pregnancy, he 'returns to the mother to finish the child'. The final penetration 'wakes the child' so it does not stay 'asleep and die inside the mother': the infusion of semen 'closes the first mouth', sealing over the fontanelle through which the foetus took in nourishment at the start of gestation. When men discuss the symbolism of flute playing or the process of actual conception and birth, they describe parallel stages of a man's 'blowing into the mother', 'withdrawing his wind (or penis)' for a marked interval and then returning to 'finish' or 'blow out the child'. But, in the secret exchange of flutes during the rites of marriage, men *perform* their procreative role as if it were a joint venture, as if it were achieved in the transmission of flute and bride from the father of the bride to the groom, in a transaction that opens the second 'vagina for bearing the child'.

Before a groom can actually play his father-in-law's instruments he, or his father, has to empty them. The father-in-law sends the flutes stuffed with pieces of salted, cooked meat which the groom is instructed to remove and feed to the bride. The meat is from a young pig or marsupial, animals men describe in this context as 'covered with hair'. The meat inside the flute is the prototype of a 'head' payment, a gift that the groom, or men of his patrilineage, will render to the lineage of the bride on behalf of each child born to the marriage. Since the marriage is typically an exchange of sisters, the gift of filled flutes is reciprocal and initiates the programme of exchange between male affines. The payments are called 'the head of the child', indicating that the 'hairy' meat ensconced in the flute represents the crown of a child's head appearing in the birth canal: by pulling the meat out of the end of the flute and placing it directly into the bride's newly-tattooed mouth, the father of the groom transfers the 'child's head' from one 'bride' to another, opening a second 'vagina' in each.

According to men's secret myth, the content of the first flute was not a child, nor the hairy crown of a child's head, but a plug of woman's pubic hair. According to myth, the first flute was made by a woman in the image of her body. Afterwards, she 'looked down at her sex' and decided to pull out her pubic hair to use as a plug or stopper when the instrument was not in use. One night her haunting music woke her brother, a small boy asleep in the men's house. He crawled to her house in the darkness, laid in wait until morning, then crept into her house and stole her flute. He did not see that the hole was closed and tried to blow into it. His lips touched his sister's hair so that whiskers began to grow around his mouth – which is why men nowadays have beards. The father has a beard tattooed on the bride, men say, 'in return' for the one her mythic counterpart planted around her brother's mouth when he stole her flute. The loss of the flute altered the sister, too, by inducing her first menstruation.

Before and during the marriage ritual, men enact various episodes of their secret myth. Weeks before the marriage, at the time the father of the bride manufactures the flutes he will fill with 'hair-covered' meat, he also has the bride's face tattooed, instructing the tattooist to repeat the designs he etched around the flutes' blowing holes. He thus recreates the mythic plug of pubic hair in various forms, in the bride's tattoos, in the flute's edible contents and in the etched decorations. Before an instrument is played for the first time, men rub the decorations with a mixture of pig fat and red pandanus oil to com-memorate the mythic removal of the plug and the onset of the first men-struation. They manufacture flutes as replicas of the brides' closed bodies and then open them through the 'secret' act of exchange, pulling out the pubic hair plug and creating a 'second vagina', a second way out. Through their trans-action, the father of the bride and the groom – who is given the 'same name' as the brother of the bride and thus stands in the symbolic relation of son to the bride's father – avoid a fatal collision: each acquires a separate orifice so that father and son, or first and second 'husbands', avert a confrontation that would cause the first menstruation, an event that represents, Gimi say, 'the death of the firstborn child'.

Once the flute passes from the father of the bride to the groom it is opened and has two 'vaginas': a blowing hole where the player inserts his 'wind' and a crying hole where the 'cries of the child' emerge. Like the pre-partum and post-partum taboos that, for most of the time, keep a man away from his pregnant and lactating wife, the two holes in the flute divide a woman's sexual and reproductive functions so that she is wife or mother but never both 'in the same hole' or at the same time. Like a flute, she has a silent lower body where a man 'goes in' and an effusive upper body where her child is carried into the world, where she holds it in her arms, produces soothing words and songs and a flow of milk. She is like the woman cited by Devereux who declared, while nursing her baby, that she felt 'sawn in two: my breasts and the upper half of my body belong to my baby, while my sexual organs and the lower half of my body belong to my husband' (Devereux, 1978: 182).

THE SECRET OF THE FLUTES ACCORDING TO WOMEN

The second Gimi theme relevant to Devereux's hypothesis is of a different order from the first. For men, the secret of the flutes is a kind of constitutional secret: men say their social and political authority and, indeed, the whole world order rest ultimately upon their keeping the flutes hidden from women. If even one woman were to see the sacred instruments – and live to speak of it – she would take them back and women would regain their autonomy. Life would lose any semblance of meaning or order: men's enemies would defeat them; gardens and pig herds would fail; seasons would falter; birds and marsupials would disappear from clan forests. According to men's secret myths and ritual practices, the flute embodies a mythic woman or a bride: why should women be forbidden to see a pristine version of themselves? In women's myths, the flute – that is, its various disguised counterparts – takes on a different identity, one that is decidedly phallic. In some myths, the flute appears as a hollow tree trunk filled with birds to represent woman's life-filled body. In others, the flute is symbolised as the giant penis of the moon or first man, piercing the night like a moonbeam or looping down, as a liana vine, from the immense height of a forest tree. When the first man was fast asleep inside his house, women's myth says, his penis awoke in the night and went out by himself to search for woman. The penis found her alone and asleep inside her house but could not penetrate her because the vagina was closed. The penis 'ate' the opening to gain entry and the woman awoke. She cut off the enormous thing that invaded her while she slept and the blood that flowed – the blood of the moon or first man – was the blood of first menses.

Men and women have different versions of how the flute got its second hole or of how woman began to menstruate. According to men's flute myth, it happened when the small boy stole his sister's flute and pulled out the plug of her pubic hair. In the matching male rite, the flute is opened not through the daring of the brother alone but through the transaction between the groom, who assumes his identity or 'same name', and the bride's father. But in women's myth, the deed is done by no man: the sister creates her own second hole or 'vagina' by cutting herself off from the first man and cutting him down to size. If men exchange sisters and flutes in order to 'reconstruct' woman's body, to separate her sexual and reproductive orifices so father and son can avoid an Oedipal collision, then, women's myth seems to add, that reconstruction can also occur with the bride's own wilful participation. But when a woman actively separates herself from the first man or father, she not only acquires a second hole or 'vagina', as it were, she makes her body into a giant penis with a bleeding 'head'.

According to the implications of men's and women's usages, marriage endows the bride with a masculine identity: she acquires a tattooed 'beard' and her body 'takes the shape' of her father's mythic severed penis. As icon of the bride or reconstructed woman, women's myths suggest as a kind of addendum, the flute is also an embodiment of the father's penis: the groom's emptying and playing the flute thus seem to enact – rather than to circumvent – a 'coital' encounter with the father of the bride. Interpreted in light of women's myths, men's exchange of women in marriage seems directly to play out what Devereux refers to as the 'homosexual triumph over the father'.

Women's myth of the giant penis makes no mention of the flute. Women allow that a menstruating woman 'cohabits with the moon, who throws his giant penis down to earth' and they acknowledge, when asked, that men call 'flute houses' the menstrual huts where women used to retire each month for the duration of their periods. Menstrual huts were also used for birthing and both sexes declare that the firstborn child – or any new infant – 'is the same as moon's blood'. But it is men who say that 'when the moon is married to a woman, when she is with her first husband (i.e., when she is menstruating), she holds the flute'. Men give explanations of flute ritual that make sense mainly in terms of the implicit content of women's myths, yet they deny that the flute is a phallic object. When I put the question directly, men reiterated that it embodied the first woman – not a penis! – as if I had failed to grasp their earlier exegeses.

The usages of each sex make explicit meanings that those of the other sex camouflage or deny. The further my analysis progressed, the more articulate women's myths seemed to become; the more they seemed to put into words unstated implications of men's ritual artefacts and actions. Analysed together, Gimi women's and men's myths and exegeses and their separate, 'secret' ritual performances can be 'read' as a multi-stranded conversation, as if each sex – while openly shunning the other – were clandestinely producing myths and rites in response to the other, to protest or alter or enlarge upon the other's versions. Gimi myths not only 'think among themselves', as Lévi-Strauss says, they also seem to dispute one another like entries in a debate over which sex ought to possess the flutes – which one provoked the first menstruation and is therefore to blame for the birth of death. Through myth and rite, men and women conduct an argument over the origin and nature of their sexual relation; and it is the shared premises of that argument – the unspoken, or half-spoken, terms upon which the sexes agree to differ – that I suggest generates the blueprint for marriage and exchange. Like the procreative beliefs of Australian Aborigines, these secretly shared yet contested fantasies about sex and procreation, about what transpires in the hidden precincts of a woman's body, 'constitute the foundation stones of their cosmogony, kinship system, religion, and social organization' (Montagu, 1974: 230).

Perhaps the most striking feature of Gimi myths of both sexes is that they delete or deactivate the father, men's myths being more emphatic in this regard, more obscure than women's myths in the way they symbolise the father's non-participation in the first marriage. In women's myth, the first man is fast asleep while his penis goes out alone. But in men's myth he is entirely missing: woman invents the flute by herself and stuffs the hole with her own pubic hair. In marriage ritual, too, fathers remain conspicuously out of sight. The fathers of the marrying pairs co-ordinate the secret phases of the rites from behind the scenes. The father of the bride goes into the forest to make new flutes from wild bamboo and fills them with meat that represents 'the head of his child'. But to send his flutes to the groom, he uses his son as intermediary, telling him to instruct the groom on how to unload them from the net bag the bride carries and how to feed the meat to the bride.

We glimpse the father, as it were, only when we consider the men's myth in the context of their rites: when we project the solitary flute-owning woman onto the figure of the bride, she becomes a kind of composite character, one whose pubic hair camouflages the hair-covered 'head of her father's child'. The father's hidden presence is like an unspeakable message that he communicates visually in the ritual representations of the flute plug – in the 'hairy' meat he hides inside the flute, in the 'pubic hair' he etches around the mouth of his flute and in the matching 'beard' he has tattooed around his daughter's mouth. The meat, the flute designs and the bride's tattoos all *show without words* that she comes to her husband as a closed instrument, one filled with her father and remade in his image.

It is women's usages that make the flute's phallic meaning explicit and thus reinforce the symbolically homosexual significance of men's traffic in women. In the combined context of women's and men's lore, the flute becomes an icon both of the bride *and* of her father's mythic penis. By endowing the bride with a beard and matching her with his flute, a man recreates his daughter as an extension of himself and in his primordial image. But the very acts by which he mythologises and masculinises the bride also fill her with 'the head of his child'. The father's transformation of the bride into a boy, or clone of himself, is also a symbolic impregnation.

The bride becomes a kind of pregnant son, in this sense. But, unlike a boy, she has no penis to collect and release her body-substance. She has no organ to discharge her father's gift and it gets stuck inside her; the child's head lodges in the birth canal and plugs her 'playing hole' so that no cries – no living child – can emerge. According to women's myth, the bride is closed for a further reason. She is enraged by her father's gift, by his installing his 'head' inside her while she was asleep and unaware, and she cuts it off as soon as she awakes. In the combined logic of men's and women's myths, unplugging the flute or bride has the meaning not only of bringing out a child but also of quelling woman's fury, of sacrificing the first child, letting it out as menstrual blood – or as 'killed' and 'hair-covered' meat – so that a second child can be born alive from a new hole. A man gives his daughter in marriage and teaches the groom how to 'play' her, in this sense, so that another man – one who has his son's 'same name' – can 'blow out' the child he installed. The men trick the bride, hiding the flutes inside her own net bag, telling her they are containers of salt, etc., so they can carry out the transaction inside her, the one installing the 'plug' or 'child's head' in the flute and the other withdrawing it. By their clandestine meeting, the father of the bride and the groom counteract the death that she – or her mythic counterpart – would prefer. When men exchange flutes and tattoo brides, and when the brides agree not to know of men's conspiracy so they will not be obliged to 'cut off the giant', the sexes seem to co-operate in enacting the homosexual premise of marriage.

The secret scenario of Gimi marriage ritual – the hidden presence of the bride's father and his conspiracy with the groom – resembles in many ways the literal process of conceiving a child. According to women and men, the 'work' of conception is performed solely by the husband who copulates many times with his wife in order to fill her womb with seminal fluid and install the child. But informants also say that repeated acts of intercourse are necessary to arrest the menstrual flow, to stop the moon's monthly visits by 'holding' him inside the woman, as if the husband had to make repeated offerings and arrange a kind of truce with the moon, who is the first man and the 'first husband'. Conception occurs when the woman dreams on the eve of the culminating act, once her womb is already well supplied with her husband's fluid. A woman who does not dream cannot conceive because only during a dream can an ancestral spirit enter her fontanelle and make its way into her womb, there 'encountering' her husband. The essential procreative moment occurs in the hidden precincts of her body when ancestor and husband – males related as father and son or grandfather and grandson – meet and come to terms.

In transacting brides, Gimi men and women seem to play out such shared fantasies. They use ritual to fill and unplug women's bodies and keep them in men's possession. When the groom (or his father) empties his father-in-law's instrument, feeds the 'hair-covered' meat to his bride and then blows into the chamber, playing his father-in-law's tune in a duet with his brother-in-law, the three men perform secret, symbolically homosexual episodes of coitus and birth that are the premise for marriage and the ensuing exchange of head payments (see Gillison, 1993).

There was a time in anthropology when myths of procreation were treated as a kind of cultural theory. In the opening pages of *The Sexual Life of Savages*, Malinowski describes the Trobriand notion that the mother contributes everything to her child as the basis for 'the rules governing descent, inheritance, succession in rank, chieftainship, hereditary offices, and magic – [of] every regulation, in fact, concerning transmission by kinship' (Malinowski, 1929: 4).

> The idea that it is solely and exclusively the mother who builds up the child's body, the man in no way contributing to its formation, is the most important factor in the legal system of the Trobrianders. (ibid.: 3)

To a Trobriand child, the father is a 'stranger', an 'outsider'; one whom the child addresses as *tama* or 'husband of my mother'. Malinowski regarded what he believed to be Trobrianders' ignorance 'of the man's share in the begetting of children' as the basis of kin terms and marriage rules (ibid.: 5–6). 'Love-making, marriage, and kinship are three aspects of the same subject,' he said (ibid.: 8).

The problem with Malinowski's hypothesis, according to his contemporaries, was that it provided little basis for systematic comparison. Notions of virgin birth, myths of insemination by ancestral spirits, were themselves irrational ideas that could hardly be used to generate stable categories. The aim of fieldwork was to produce descriptions of societies that would make them comparable because '[w]ithout classification', Radcliffe-Brown said, 'there can be no science' (1964: 2). In place of indigenous misconceptions about where babies come from, British functionalists used residence rules, kin terms and the linearity of descent to create typologies and move the study of social structure onto what they held to be a higher, more theoretical plane.

Procreation beliefs were not merely fantastic and irrational. They were also graphically sexual. Considered as 'the foundation stones of . . . social organization' (Montagu, 1974: 230), they created the unacceptable impression that savages devised rules governing 'descent, inheritance, succession in rank', etc., on the basis of sexual fantasies; and hence that they actually believed their fantasies and were deficient natural historians, ignorant of the facts of life – a conclusion that sounded supercilious and racist (Leach, 1967). But an explanation already existed that took account of the ethnographic data without insinuating an insulting ignorance. In 1925 Ernest Jones suggested that the father's role is disguised and denied rather than unknown.

> The father disappears from the scene only to reappear in a disguised form. The idea of the powerful and hated father is sacrificed in favour of an ancestral spirit, who in a supernatural manner impregnates the mother; for both the Australian ratapas and the Trobriand waiwais

emanate from ancestors, and no one who has had the opportunity of analysing a member of an ancient English family or an American with a passion for genealogy can fail to discover that forefathers are psychologically nothing but fathers at a slight remove. (Jones, 1925: 122)

But anthropologists dismissed the relevance of any psychoanalytic theory of unconscious thought and repression and continued for years to debate the sexual ignorance of savages, arguing over whether Trobriand Islanders or Australian Aborigines indeed failed to grasp the 'fertilizing agency of the male seed' (Spiro, 1968: 248); whether they actually believed, as Austin reported of Trobrianders, that the 'man's contribution towards the new life in the mother's body was nil' (cited in Spiro, 1968). Anthropologists refused to consider the fact that, at the same time as Trobriand informants emphatically denied the father's role, their myths and procreation beliefs gave dramatic evidence of a precise – although concealed – understanding of the male function (Malinowski, 1929). What Trobrianders were 'ignoring', it seems to me extrapolating from Gimi data, was not the contribution of the male but the presence of the father – in addition to the husband.

In terms of their articulated views, Gimi appear in striking contrast to the classic aboriginal. Gimi men and women assert that a husband's semen forms the whole child and that a woman's body is merely the receptacle. But in denying the mother's active role, Gimi seem really to deny the hidden presence of her father – his entry through the fontanelle in a dream – and thereby hide the alliance of husband's semen and father's blood. What they deny, in other words, is the homosexual connection between men that is the final cause of life. From this point of view, Trobrianders' insistence upon the primacy of ancestral spirit in causing conception achieves the same end by an opposite tactic: whereas Gimi dismiss the spirit-father or moon or mythic giant (or, in the terms of marriage ritual, the father of the bride), Trobrianders and Australian Aboriginals sacrifice the living penetrator in favour of a disembodied ancestor. Each underestimates or 'gets rid' of *one* of the men who penetrates woman's body and thereby conceals their homosexual relation.

If Gimi rules of kinship and marriage indeed enact such tacit beliefs, they suggest that a symbolic male homosexuality lies at the core of Gimi social organisation in much the way Devereux proposed. Looked at in this light, exchanges of sisters and head payments are a means to subvert men's sexual aims by carrying them out in substitute form, a means to counteract yet achieve the unspeakable secrets implied in the debate between men's and women's myths. To the degree that Gimi women adopt, both in public ritual and in secret rites of their own, the male identity that marriage imposes, they seem to collude with men in achieving men's aims.

-- note begins --

NOTE

1 The fieldwork upon which this article is based was carried out mainly in Ubagubi, a village of Gimi-speaking people in the Eastern Highlands of Papua New Guinea, and covers a span of a dozen years. My work began in 1973–4 with twenty months in the field, followed in 1975 by a further six-month stay, and then continued, in the form of intermittent summer visits of three to four months, until 1985. The impetus for my original research among the Gimi was to describe the society from a female point of view, to use women's own accounts, life histories, attitudes to men, etc., to portray the lives of both sexes; but my work expanded to include men's views (see Gillison, 1993).

During the period of fieldwork I was married to David Gillison, a photographer and rainforest conservationist. Accounts of events that transpired inside men's houses are compilations of reports by Gimi men of four initiations that occurred during the period of fieldwork. Many informants' comments and explanations were inspired by tape-recordings made during the proceedings by David Gillison.

BIBLIOGRAPHY

Delaney, C. (1986) 'The meaning of paternity and the virgin birth debate', *Man* ns 21: 494–513.

Devereux, G. (1978) 'Ethnopsychoanalytic reflections on the notion of kinship (1965)', in *Ethnopsychoanalysis: Psychoanalysis and Anthropology as Complementary Frames of Reference*. Berkeley: University of California Press.

Douglas, M. (1970) *Purity and Danger: An Analysis of Concepts of Pollution and Taboo*. Harmondsworth: Pelican.

Durkheim, E. (1985 [1966]) *The Rules of Sociological Method*. New York: The Free Press.

Evans-Pritchard, E. E. (1965) *Theories of Primitive Religion*. Oxford: Clarendon Press.

Freud, S. (1976 [1900]) *The Interpretation of Dreams*, trans. J. Strachey. Harmondsworth: Pelican.

Gajdusek, D. C. (1970) *Diaries, 1959–70*. Mimeo. National Institute of Health. Bethesda, Maryland.

Gillison, G. (1993) *Between Culture and Fantasy: A New Guinea Highlands Mythology*. Chicago: University of Chicago Press.

Herdt, G. H. (1981) *Guardians of the Flutes*. New York: McGraw-Hill.

Jones, E. (1925) 'Mother-right and the sexual ignorance of savages', *International Journal of Psycho-Analysis* 6: 109–30.

Kelly, R. C. (1976) 'Witchcraft and sexual relations: an exploration in the social and semantic implications of the structure of belief', in P. Brown and G. Buchbinder (eds) *Man and Woman in the New Guinea Highlands*. Special Publication no. 8. Washington, DC: American Anthropological Association.

Langness, L. L. (1974) 'Ritual, power and male dominance in the New Guinea Highlands', *Ethos* 2: 189–212.

Leach, E. R. (1967) 'Virgin birth', *Proceedings of the Royal Anthropological Institute for 1966*: 39–50.

Lévi-Strauss, C. (1969 [1949]) *The Elementary Structures of Kinship*, trans. J. H. Bell, J. R. von Strumer and R. Needham. Boston: Beacon Press.

224 Working models

—— (1977) *L'Identité: Seminaire Dirigé Par Claude Lévi-Strauss*. Quadrige: Presses Universitaires de France.

—— (1988) *The Jealous Potter*, trans. B. Chorier. Chicago and London: University of Chicago Press.

Malinowski, B. (1929) *The Sexual Life of Savages in North-Western Melanesia*. London: Routledge.

Mauss, M. (1967) *The Gift: Forms and Functions of Exchange in Archaic Societies*, trans. I. Cunnison. New York: Norton.

Montagu, M. F. A. (1974) *Coming into Being among the Australian Aborigines*. London: Routledge & Kegan Paul. Cited in Delaney, 1986.

Radcliffe-Brown, A. R. (1964) 'Introduction', in A. R. Radcliffe-Brown and D. Forde (eds) *African Systems of Kinship and Marriage*. London: Oxford University Press.

Read, K. E. (1952) 'Nama cult of the Central Highlands, New Guinea', *Oceania* 23: 1–25.

—— (1965) *The High Valley*. New York: Scribner's.

Salisbury, R. F. (1965) 'The Siane of the Eastern Highlands', in P. Lawrence and M. J. Meggitt (eds) *Gods, Ghosts and Men in Melanesia*. Melbourne: Oxford University Press.

Schiefflin, E. L. (1976) *The Sorrow of the Lonely and the Burning of the Dancers*. New York: St Martin's Press.

Spiro, M. E. (1968) 'Virgin birth, parthenogenesis, and physiological paternity: an essay on cultural interpretation', *Man* ns 3: 242–61.

Williams, F. E. (1969 [1936]) *Papuans of the Trans-Fly*. Oxford: Oxford University Press.

14 Psychoanalysis as content
Reflections on Chapters 11, 12 and 13

R. H. Hook

It was suggested in Chapter 7 that it might be useful to distinguish between the process of psychoanalysis and its other aspects, there summarily labelled 'content', without any attempt to characterise content, though content would have to include at least some account of what people think, feel and do, how they behave and respond: the findings of psychoanalysis. Another aspect of psychoanalysis would have to do with formulations about the 'structure' of the mind, metapsychology, allied inevitably to its metaphysics, i.e., its ontology and epistemology. These three aspects of psychoanalysis, process, content and structure, will be found to be interrelated but in what way they are interrelated is beyond the scope of this paper.

Obviously a great deal has been known about human responses and behaviour and for a very long time, though what is known may be repeatedly lost: denied, repressed, forgotten or simply ignored, only to be rediscovered at a later time. I am referring of course to what great thinkers, writers and artists have known about and dealt with. Freud himself quoted extensively from the work of earlier writers and artists. The list in James Strachey's *Standard Edition* of the 'works of painting and sculpture, music, drama, poetry, fiction, as well as some myths, legends and fairy tales' quoted or discussed by Freud runs to over seven pages and contains several hundred entries (*S.E.* 24: 187–94). Such material would not have been so ready to hand had not the 'content' of the mind already been largely known and also common property. Lévi-Strauss makes essentially the same point:

> At every step, or almost every step, we met notions and categories, in perfectly explicit form – such as those of the oral and anal character – which psychoanalysts cannot claim to have discovered: they have done no more than rediscover them.
>
> Better still, *Totem and Taboo* complete was anticipated in a significant advance by the Jivaro Indians in the myth which for them takes the place of *Genesis*. . . . From a psychological perspective the plot of the

Jivaro myth appears even more rich and subtle than that of *Totem and Taboo*. (Lévi-Strauss, 1985: 243–4, my translation)

Though denying any primacy to the *'code psycho-organique'* (which psychoanalysts discover in the early stages of thinking, and especially in primary process thinking), Lévi-Strauss elegantly displays in his structural analyses the sort of psychic content with which psychoanalysts have become increasingly familiar. What Freud demonstrated was just how basic to thinking and behaviour such content is. Content came to be equated with psychoanalysis. The Oedipus complex is a case in point: revolutionary when first promulgated, it is now widely accepted, as the above quotation from Lévi-Strauss implies, while the concept itself has been extended to include earlier stages of development.[1]

In passing we might note an interesting point raised by the above quotation from Lévi-Strauss: who did discover the Oedipus complex? Was it Oedipus (or his real-life equivalent); was it Sophocles, who gave it dramatic form; was it Freud, who formulated the theory; or was it the Jivaro, whose mythology is 'even more rich and subtle'? The early Christians believed in God the Father, they believed Jesus was the Son of God, they believed in the Holy Spirit; did they believe in a Triune God, or was that only possible after the doctrine of the Trinity had been enunciated? Isn't it a matter of the difference between knowing *p* and *knowing that p*: recognising something, naming it and putting it into propositional form where it can be discussed, asserted, denied, tested and so forth? When there is a readily available concept or category, things or events may be recognised as belonging to it and the capacity to perceive or apprehend is extended. 'Oedipus' as a 'complex' of mental events would not have been recognised by the Jivaro even though the recorded occurrences themselves might not have seemed strange. There is a great difference between operating a myth at the primary process level and formulating it in secondary process, logical, terms.

The three preceding chapters in this section, 'Working models', offer accounts of different ways in which Oedipal phantasies may be expressed in the myths and rituals of different societies. Suzette Heald and L. R. Hiatt raise questions about the applicability of classical psychoanalytic views to their material while Gillian Gillison integrates psychoanalytic concepts into her account and makes explanation in terms of the unconscious part of her explanation of cultural phenomena.

CIRCUMCISION AND THE PRIMAL FATHER

In 'Indulgent fathers and collective male violence', Hiatt poses what at first sight appears to be a problem, and implies, in effect, that psychoanalytic theory may need to be revised: if the archetypal father of *Totem and Taboo* is 'a violent male who defends his harem against all-comers and drives out his sons as they reach puberty', how are we to account for the evident reality of paternal love, seen for instance in the case of Aka fathers nursing their infants, or Australian Aboriginal fathers interacting with their offspring and rebuking the mothers for unnecessary harshness, and at the time of circumcision expressing sympathy for their sons and directing their resentment of the ill-treatment of the boys towards the women? A similar question is asked by Heald in 'Every man a hero', when comparing the roles of Gisu fathers and mothers in infant care and at the time of circumcision. When a Gisu boy is suddenly and violently weaned it is his father who offers protection and threatens the mother, the boy's classificatory sister offering 'sexual services' to comfort and reassure. Heald too challenges the traditional, *Totem and Taboo* view of circumcision: 'Gisu circumcision [presenting] itself initially as a striking negative example', and asks, by implication, How would a psychoanalyst today deal with *this* material?

Does not the difficulty lie in the assumption that the behaviour of the 'archetypal father of *Totem and Taboo*' (were he to have existed) would be definitive of all subsequent paternal behaviour? This would be to expect too much of the theory; nor is it clear that it is what Freud intended: what Freud offered was an explanation of certain features common to dreams, neurotic behaviour and the myths and rituals of primitive societies, especially in relation to the phenomena of totemism and associated taboos. It would also imply a very determinist view of human behaviour, accounting for the social present, down to the details of the behaviour of fathers towards their male offspring, in terms of an event, or series of events, occurring in the remote past.

The Oedipus story does not of course require a violent archetypal father (if anything, it implies, rather, violence on the part of the son), though the 'primal parricide' of *Totem and Taboo* does; what the Oedipus situation entails is ambivalence of the male child towards his father, wishing to be rid of him so that he can possess his mother exclusively,[2] a state of affairs which once existed and with the loss of which he has already had to struggle. This close, narcissistic, encompassing relationship between infant and nursing (or pregnant) mother arouses father's jealousy and envy. To a degree, in patrilineal societies at least, the envy of the father may be mitigated by identification with his son as his heir and successor who will eventually replace him – a circumstance which may carry a certain survival value in helping to control filicidal impulses.

We have in effect a triangular situation: the child envies the combined parents in a relationship from which he is excluded (Oedipus); the father envies the child's close bond with the mother; and the mother no doubt (later) envies her son as he is taken off to the men's world of ritual and power from which she is excluded, as well, it might be added, as possessing the penis and all that implied. For the moment however we are concerned with the first of these relationships.

The myth of the Rainbow Serpent, in which hostility of the son towards the father is clear enough, highlighting the transition to manhood of Tjiniman and the displacement of Kanmanggur, has obvious primary process characteristics: Tjiniman omnipotently repairs his broken bones and has a good sleep; he cuts his nose and repairs the wound, that is, circumcises himself (nose = penis), a (manic) assertion of autonomy and control and a denial of passivity, neediness and dependence (depressive): 'It wasn't done *to* me; I did it to myself'. In this way he deals also with feelings of abandonment precipitated by the ritual – which formally separated him from his mother's care: he complains, 'no one looked after me'. On returning to the camp his father welcomes him but, 'in a language no one understands' (the intrusion of ambiguity, concealing and revealing: language is for communicating; a language 'no one understands' is for not communicating), Tjiniman says, 'I am going to kill your father', but then, no one took revenge, no one mourned Kanmanggur and Tjiniman's deed was not execrated. Kanmanggur, the primal father, is now replaced by Tjiniman, the son, representing the 'horde of brothers', the successors.

Clearly we are in the world of dream and myth where even horrific events may occur without any appropriate accompanying emotional response: no shock or horror is recorded. The similarity between myth and dream hardly needs emphasis. In both, what is similar is identical: the serpent and the pottery jar (Jivaro myth) need no interpreting; one hollow object, one long or extensible, tubular object, can stand for another, can indeed *be* that other. A thing may be represented by its complement or by its opposite, by a part, or by a similar or associated object – some of the mechanisms of 'symmetric' logic operating in transformations in both myth and dream. In the deeper layers of the mind isomorphism becomes identity and the distinction between inside and outside is non-existent.[3]

Noting Stanner's polemic against *Totem and Taboo*, Hiatt quotes him in words which it would also be possible to construe as implying that the myth did record the forgotten parricide: 'For here is a myth standing alone as though it were a monument to something forgotten but vaguely familiar, and rife with suggestive silences.' Or is it a monument to a universal *phantasy* parricide, repeated in every generation? Tjiniman climbs a cliff face by means of a rope which is cut or breaks; Lévi-Strauss quotes similar material in myths from South America; the 'Song of Bolia' (Chapter 3) refers to a chain suspended from the sky which is climbed; 'Jacob's Ladder' and 'Jack and the Beanstalk' are similar. How is it that some themes are so widespread, if not indeed universal? Are these only about erections? Why is belief in another world, above or below, so prevalent? Is it a search for an ideal, or idealised, but now lost, past experience? Or does the 'other world' reflect a partial awareness of another (internal) world – where extraordinary things happen? Should we not seek the origin and meaning of these – and of parricide too – in universal themes of primary process phantasy?

The Rainbow Serpent, Angamunggi, the primeval Father, is androgynous (like many creator gods), 'has a womb and once gave birth to a son' – a somewhat less improbable story than that of Adam's rib, or Athena springing fully armed from the head of Zeus. Anatomical details, like time and space, may be distorted or ignored in dream and myth, though later, in secondary revision or under interrogation, they may be added or corrected: a body space, an 'inside', a 'container', is enough; mother's body contains 'other babies', or 'spirit children', or whatever. The universal mother is also the devouring mother, Karwadi, embodying oral phantasies of eating or being eaten, of incorporating or being incorporated, and annihilation.

Ambivalence pervades this series of myths. In the 'Circumcision Rite', acceptance of society's demands coexists with hostility towards society and its rules: 'The escort party dramatically announces its return by throwing a ceremonial spear into the centre of the home community's circle of camp fires . . . the boy's close kin give forth with lamentations' – showing identification of the brothers-in-law with the initiates' suppressed anger and hostility and giving expression also to the emotions dominating the rival groups and the ambivalence of the struggle being played out between them, especially between the boy and his mother, and between the men and the women, an ambivalence seen also in the Bullroarer Rite which celebrates masculinity and potency: the women are shouldered aside, the boys turn their backs on their mothers, becoming, like dingo pups, 'tamed', as they enter the world of men, of camaraderie and good humour, of 'singing and moving in unison, [with] high levels of body contact, and periodic euphoria', the world of moral homosexuality – also reinforcing control and supplanting aggression.

The stark contrast invoked by Hiatt is only apparent. At the primary process level there is no incompatibility: the hated and murdered father, envied, dreaded and experienced as threatening, is also the loving and caring father, revered and respected. As maturity proceeds the two sides of the ambivalence can be better accepted and the father more nearly seen for what he in fact is and always has been. In myth and dream some aspects are split off and projected.

Behind these events lies the problem of reconciling the fundamental ambivalences inherent in all human relationships: one pole of the ambivalence being given free rein, and even augmented, while (and because) the other is repressed or displaced. This polarity was characterised by Freud in the dualism of the life and death instincts (or 'drives' – *lebenstriebe, todestriebe*). Criticism, especially of the latter concept, is directed towards the difficulty of finding a physiological base for such an instinct but the problem really arises from the use of a term which in English has an unambiguous biological reference, absent from, or at least qualified in, the original German: that there is such a polarity between what is constructive and what is destructive in human affairs can hardly be doubted.

In 'Every man a hero', Heald places the emphasis on that deployment and control of aggression through which the boy ostensibly becomes a man: he demonstrates that he can be aggressive, indeed in effect violent towards himself without showing fear, and able to control not only his fear but his aggression too. The idea of being 'caught by the ancestral power of circumcision' reifies power, and personifies circumcision as possessing and transmitting power, the power of the ancestors, now descended on the boy. Heald's analysis brings out the ambivalence attaching to the concept of *lirima* which, at least in part, reflects or expresses this power. Usually representing the 'negative' emotions of envy, jealousy, hatred, resentment and shame and seen as responsible for all the trouble in the community, *lirima* acquires 'positive' value in circumcision, and is necessary for war. Rather than inducing *lirima*, which is the function of the preparatory ritual, the circumcision cuts themselves seem to be a token of its presence, making it manifest.

Does not the 'meaning' of the Gisu circumcision ritual then lie in the socialising of aggressive impulses rather than in coping with, as classically represented, erotic (Oedipal) impulses and symbolising the power of the father, reinforcing the incest taboo. In the Gisu case, the power of the father appears to be displaced on to the ancestors, and the Oedipal conflict resolved, at least outwardly, when the boy becomes mature and acquires a wife. The power of the father is real only before circumcision and until then rivalry exists mainly on a fantasy level; after that it can be realised, and in Gisu society apparently often is, openly and even violently in parricide and filicide.

Quoting Wangusa's novel, Heald suggests a link between violent weaning and circumcision rituals. The loss of the mother – the idealised 'good breast' – is the introduction to what Melanie Klein called the 'depressive position'. When the loss of the good object cannot be tolerated and accepted, the lost good object, instead of being in phantasy introjected and symbolised (considered to be the beginning of symbolism), is split and projected, normal progress is blocked and pathological psychotic processes dominate. Ambivalence towards mother is obvious in the quotation from Wangusa: '*Mother-bad-good-bad-good-why?*' – pointing to the splitting and coexistence of phantasy 'good' and 'bad' mothers in conflict and in the process of being internalised, or projected. Gisu ritual mirrors unconscious aggressive phantasies and the variations through which these are played out, offering expression to and reinforcement of attempted solutions.

AMBIVALENCE AND AMBIGUITY

Heald's material illustrates also the element of ambivalence or ambiguity in destructive violence: death linked to life, 'Unless a seed of wheat fall to the ground and die, it cannot live' (Biblical proverb). The fermenting, bubbling up of the yeast in the making of ritual beer is linked to the bubbling up of *lirima*. 'You have spoilt it!': the 'spoiling', of the yeast, of defloration, of circumcision, all seem to relate to the notion of a pristine, but impotent, innocence, like that lost by eating of the fruit of the Tree of Knowledge, the forbidden fruit of the Garden of Eden, but needing to be lost or spoiled before movement forward can proceed.

The equating symbolically of sexuality and numerous other activities and processes – ploughing fields, making war, manufacturing pots, brewing beer – has long been recognised; hence the need for sexual abstinence during the course of these activities lest they be diminished and spoilt, or enhanced ('too strong'). Psychoanalytic theory recognises that there is in all sexuality a degree of fusion of libido (*eros*) and aggression (*thanatos*).

Ambiguity stands out in 'Symbolic homosexuality and cultural theory'. Do they know, or do they not know? Ambiguity about knowing and not knowing is one of the features of primary process thinking: Gimi – and other – men and women both 'know' and 'do not know' at the same time. This is what makes myth, religion and art captivating: it enables people to deal in things they both know and do not know, or are not permitted or expected to know. It also contributes to the idea of myth and dream as communicating 'secret messages' and psychoanalysis as hermeneutic. Take for instance John Steiner's (1985, 1990) discussion of the drama of Oedipus: Oedipus behaved as though ignorant of what he was actually in a very good position to know; Jocasta's self-reproach (and also that of Oedipus) was really based on being faced with the consequences of what had been known all along, but ignored, distorted or denied. Consider also Gillison's data: Gimi men know 'the facts of life', but operate a ritual which explicitly denies what they implicitly know. Reality is not just evaded, it is actively misrepresented and distorted. How conscious or unconscious is this distortion? Ambiguity and ambivalence are characteristic of bi-logical thinking and follow from the interpenetration of primary and secondary process.

How far we have come from the notion of a 'fixed' symbolism:

According to men's secret myths and ritual practices, the flute embodies both a mythic woman or a bride*. . . . In women's myths, the flute – that is, its various disguised counterparts – takes on a different identity, one that is decidedly phallic. In some myths, the flute appears as a hollow tree trunk filled with birds [both recognizable phallic symbols] to represent woman's life-filled body. In others, the flute is symbolised as the giant penis of the moon or first man.

[* with the suppressed equation, flute = penis, penis embodies 'mythic woman and bride', a double representation characteristic of 'symmetric' logic]

What we see here is an example of the flexibility, the overdetermined nature and the ambiguity of primary process symbolic thinking, identity of part and whole ('part-object' penis = 'whole object' woman and bride), identity by association and by similarity, and 'magical' (i.e., omnipotent) thinking: 'His lips (labia) touched his sister's hair so that whiskers (pubic hair) began to grow around his mouth. . . . The loss of the flute altered the sister, too, by inducing her first menstruation.'

Take another quotation from Gillison's paper:

his penis awoke in the night and went out by himself to search for woman . . . but could not penetrate her because the vagina was closed. The penis 'ate' the opening to gain entry and the woman awoke

which seems to allude to the state of pre-pubescence and later deflowering: 'the blood of the moon or first man – was the blood of first menses' (and also of the ruptured hymen?) links menstrual periodicity with the phases of the moon; i.e., controlled by the moon, the first man, viz., women's sexuality is controlled by men. If the elements of myth represent primary process phantasies, as I believe they do, we may see in myths an external representation of basic patterns of thinking and mental content, which, being externalised and in that way made more objective, may be more convincing than psychoanalysts' reports of dream material. Here we have an example of primary process mental content and of bi-logical thinking: viz. a 'part-object' penis and its representation in a personification (mental institutions are frequently represented in this way) with power of independent action, and having projected into it an oral aggressive impulse: 'the penis "ate" the opening to gain entry'.

PSYCHOANALYSIS AND ANTHROPOLOGY

To come back to psychoanalysis and the study of culture and society, Heald asks whether the coming together of the two perspectives, ethnographic and psychoanalytic, will give a determinate understanding of either, raising questions about what a determinate answer would be, and indeed how it would be established that a given account was determinate, in the sense, presumably, of 'settled, fixed and unlikely to vary'. The expectations of psychoanalysts and anthropologists were raised by Freud's claim to give a 'determinate' account both of mind and of the origins of society and culture – in an original parricide, or series of repeated parricides.

Discussing Freud's metapsychology, Michael Moore commented: 'Freud viewed his metapsychology as justified by its ability to relate mind to brain. From the unpublished "Project" of 1895 . . . to the *Outline [of Psycho-Analysis]* . . . he first and last saw his task as building a theory to relate brain to mind' (1988: 153–4). We might propose another question in a similar form to Heald's: would the bringing together of the two perspectives of psychoanalysis and brain physiology make possible a determinate account of either? Initially at least, Freud thought it would and set out to give an account of mind in terms of brain physiology, hence his early schema of permeable and impermeable neurones, quantities of excitation, etc. (Freud, 1950 [1895]: 295), and the continuing role of energy (libido and its cathexis) in his theoretical formulations.

Whatever is concluded about the relation between mental events and brain states, it is unlikely that either will be found to be reducible without residues to the other. Such a reduction is neither possible nor desirable: to account for mind solely in terms of brain states would effectively eliminate mind – as constituted in specifically 'mental' events. Similarly to give an account of mind in societal terms or of society in terms only of mind, were either possible, would be to replace either set of terms by the other, and our understanding of both would be impoverished. It is only when they are recognised as separate and equally real that the relations between them can be properly studied.

Freud's thesis of *Totem and Taboo* rests at least partially on the recapitulation theory of human development, of ontogeny repeating phylogeny. If a determinate account of the *origins* of mind and culture were to be possible would it not have to be in terms of an event separate from either? Culture, language, mind, brain (and perhaps other features of human anatomy as well) appear to have evolved in mutual interaction, but what precipitated this course of development in hominid evolution is not known. Genetic mutation and selection, including a genic representation for altruism, has been suggested by Badcock (1980: 33) in a recent attempt to pursue this line of enquiry.

It is reasonable to think that there is an ongoing developmental interaction between culture and mind. Even the development, as a cultural phenomenon, of psychoanalysis itself seems to have brought about some change in personality patterns and the mode of presentation of neurosis: the early methods of psychoanalysis, once apparently effective in removing hysterical symptoms quite quickly, no longer seem to work in the same way today; analyses are longer – perhaps precisely for the reason that the types of personality disturbance now seen by psychoanalysts have changed.

Addressing the question, how should an anthropologist use psycho-analysis?, Heald suggests that psychoanalysis has thrown a metaphorical spanner into the Durkheimian works, in that what might otherwise have been a relatively straightforward understanding of cultural symbolism has become confounded by the appearance of distorting forces, making conscious symbolism a mask for something else and 'turn[ing] our accepted interpretative canons upside-down'. Is it upside-down, or inside-out – to reveal the 'seamy' side? Heald is unable to decide about psychoanalysis: was Ricoeur then right, and psychoanalysis a hermeneutic, deciphering hidden messages concealed in symbolic guise? She seems also to suspect that somewhere there might exist an empirical base: 'the unconscious dynamic must have some external corre-lative', and concedes that 'the psychoanalytic model here frequently has an alternative mode of validation . . . in its therapeutic claims'. I think the signifi-cant fact that Heald is alluding to here is that the analysand can respond to the analyst in a way in which it would be impossible for a culture or a society to respond to an anthropologist (or, *a fortiori*, an historian) whose interpretations can be corrected only by further examination of the material or by bringing fresh evidence, whereas the analyst has in addition the response of the analysand and the consequential development of the material as a source of confirmation.

Parkin (Chapter 4) suggests that the association of dancing with coitus is intuitively plausible but undemonstrable. What *is* demonstrable is that rhythmic movement, or any feature common to two different ideas, may be taken by unconscious phantasy (using symmetric logic) to link, or equate, the two ideas in which it appears; what may be not demonstrable is application in a given case. Parkin's political explanation is also undemonstrable, though totally plausible, and I think this is what Heald is getting at when she talks about 'the pot calling the kettle black'. The problem clearly is to isolate and validate causal factors. Change during the course of an analysis is observable, but 'therapeutic success' is a blunderbuss and not specific enough to validate theory. Therapeutic efficacy, though supportive, cannot be decisive; nor can therapeutic failure invalidate psychoanalytic propositions.

We are right to infer an interaction between mental and social events: 'From a psychoanalytic perspective, unconscious sexual fantasies acquire a determining role in the organisation of social institutions like kinship and marriage.' Myths about flutes are used for 'political' ends, viz., validation of power and control of women – and the universe: 'indeed the whole world order rests upon a secret surrounding bamboo flutes'. We saw in Chapter 7 that a political institution, the Communist Party or the Mafia, can serve to reinforce unconscious psychological defences. In Gillison's material we see defences against the unconscious fear of women; defences protect also against the chaos of the internal world, here projected on to the external 'whole world order', held in place by the myth.

Social events are in some form also mental events and all mental events occur in a social milieu; but how are they to be connected? Devereux pointed out that any discipline cannot take the explanation of a given phenomenon beyond a certain point, the point at which another form of explanation must take over and which constitutes the partition between the two disciplines, or types of explanation. Complementarity implies that answers may be only partial and that complementary explanations come closer to a, in practice impossible, complete account. Consistently applied however, complementarity would mean that psychological and socio-logical explanations ran along parallel lines and never met. Whether or not this is so may depend upon how the material is selected and dealt with. While Parkin's material is susceptible to both political and psychological explanations, Gillison has selected and presented her material in an inte-grating way that entails both a psychoanalytic and a cultural explanation – what Devereux called an 'ethnopsychoanalytic' interpretation.[4]

In Gillison's account, observations are sited at, or from, the mind–culture partition, the point/instant of partition, where reciprocal interaction may become the subject of observation (as described by Devereux);[5] other relevant partitions are those between unconscious–conscious, at which psychoanalysis specifically sites its own interpretations, and between indi-vidual and group psychology. Gillison's material may be taken by way of illustration – and here our immediate interest is not in the validity of Devereux's psychoanalytic account of ritual homosexuality nor in Gillison's ethnographic data but in the way in which they are combined:

> The moment 'certain general psychological and cultural facts' are com-bined . . . the exchange of women in marriage [cultural phenomenon] expresses not merely the law of talion [bivalent: cultural *and* psycho-logical] or a system of *prestations mutuelles* [cultural] . . . but 'an obsessional tendency toward "*bilanisme*" . . . a compulsive quest for symmetry' [psychological] that is the hallmark of latent male homo-sexuality [psychological analysis with consequences for culture].

Here we encounter the partition mental/cultural: a reciprocal relationship between sets of 'raw facts', the cultural phenomena and hypothesised mental events and, finally, an interpretation which exemplifies and illu-minates a psychological proposition.

The institution of marriage [cultural] repels 'the threatening specter of latent homosexuality' [psychological] by allowing men to achieve their goal in symbolic form, disguising homosexuality 'as a heterosexual act',

illustrating the interaction of culture and phantasy and extending our perception of the functions of marriage.

Gimi flutes are called 'birds' and men keep them in the rafters of their club houses, forbidding women and children to see them on pain of death.

This straightforward factual statement is full of significance from an ethnopsychoanalytic point of view: that they are called 'birds', when they are not birds but flutes, draws attention to a psychological significance which might be deduced from the symbolism of birds. This, so far as it goes, presents a problem for psychological analysis; but when 'forbidding women and children to see them on pain of death' is added, so is another dimension, a cultural one, the threat of death. But the threat of death, a social dimension, is also a mental one and reinforces the symbolic significance of what is entailed in the flutes being called 'birds'.

AMBIGUITY: KNOWING AND NOT KNOWING

It doesn't matter whether we talk about Oedipus or the homosexuality of the Gimi. Do the Gimi know that a symbolic male homosexuality is at the basis of their social organisation, as Gillison suggests it is? If they do not in some way *know* it, how do they come to operate it, how could it have arisen, and why? If confronted, they would without doubt deny it as they deny that the flute is a phallic object – and that in spite of the fact that their explanations make sense mainly in terms of women's myths, in which it is.

We are now in a position to note a final ambiguity in Gillison's material. Dismissing the relevance of psychoanalysis:

Anthropologists refused to consider the fact that, at the same time as Trobriand informants emphatically denied the father's role, their myths and procreation beliefs gave dramatic evidence of a precise – although concealed – understanding of the male function.

So far so good, but,

Gimi men and women assert that a husband's semen forms the whole child and that a woman's body is merely the receptacle. But *in denying the mother's active role*, Gimi seem really to deny the hidden presence of her father [and] the homosexual connection between men that is the final cause of life. (My emphasis)

Here again we have the phantasy of container and contained: the 'container' (woman) is assigned a totally passive role – a common enough fantasy – and the 'contained', man (here as part-object, penis), becomes the sole creator – in line with a widespread mythology which embraces both *Pallas Athena* and Adam.

Are we not now confronted with a problem similar to that of knowledge about the father's role, from which we started? What do Gimi *really* know about the mother's role in reproduction? When an Australian aboriginal woman associates quickening with the arrival of the spirit child in her womb and identifies the place where it occurred as that child's country, does she know that the quickening is only the first movement of the foetus? When does 'knowledge' give place to 'myth'? In one sense, it doesn't matter. That aspect of reality which does not fit with mythology will be ignored: internal reality replaces external reality (Freud, 1915: 187).

The material of these papers has been considered mainly in terms of content but it is clear that a particular model of the mind is invoked and in this essay an attempt has been made to illustrate its essential features: unconscious mental process and content, mechanisms like projective identification, condensation, displacement and denial, and the idea of a different kind of thinking, appropriate to phantasy and symbolic trans-formations, with distortion of space and time, absence of contradiction and negation, logical connection represented by simultaneity, and causality by succession, characteristic of what Freud called 'primary process', and Matte-Blanco, 'symmetrical logic'; and to show how unconscious phantasy and culture reciprocally interact. Primary process phantasy underlies and interpenetrates not only neurotic symptoms and psychotic thinking but most, if not all, human activities, including especially myth making, religion, literature and art. It is suggested that this or a similar concept of mind may be found useful, even essential, to the understanding of culture and society and to the further development of ethnopsychoanalysis as a discipline differentiated from psychoanalysis and perhaps from anthro-pology too, though drawing on the findings of both.

NOTES

1 Cf. Britton *et al.* (1989) *The Oedipus Complex Today.*
2 Stated in more general terms, what the Oedipus situation implies is desire for removal of the parent of the same sex in order to possess the parent of the opposite sex. This is the Oedipus complex in its positive form. In its negative form it represents a desire for the parent of the same sex and removal of the parent of the opposite sex; while the inverse form consists in identification with the parent of the opposite sex in becoming the object of the desire of the parent of the same sex (cf. Freud, 1923: 33–4).

3 'Deep down the Freudian concept of symbol reflects the simultaneous expression of the separation and at the same time the identity between the symbol and
what it symbolizes' (Matte-Blanco, 1988: 242). Without a theory of the irrational elements in thinking myths cannot be understood. If it is not to be totally
meaningless, primary process thinking must necessarily follow some rules,
though obviously these are not the rules of ordinary logic.
4 Ethnopsychoanalysis, in my view, is not a felicitous term, as it implies that a
culture can be psychoanalysed, which it cannot; but it is the only one available
to denote the conjunction of psychoanalytic and ethnological concepts.
5 Devereux, 1967: Chapter 22. My use of Devereux's partition theory does not do
justice to his analysis: there are many important aspects of complementarity and
relativity, especially in regard to observation, that I have necessarily ignored.

BIBLIOGRAPHY

Badcock, C. R. (1980) *The Psychoanalysis of Culture*. Oxford: Blackwell.
Britton, R. *et al.* (1989) *The Oedipus Complex Today: Clinical Implications*.
London: Karnac.
Devereux, G. (1967) *From Anxiety to Method in the Behavioral Sciences*. The
Hague and Paris: Mouton.
Freud, S. (1950 [1895]) 'Project for a Scientific Psychology', *S.E.* 1: 283–397.
—— (1913) *Totem and Taboo, S.E.* 13: 1–162.
—— (1915) 'The unconscious', *S.E.* 14: 161–215.
—— (1923) *The Ego and the Id, S.E.* 19: 3–66.
Lévi-Strauss, C. (1985) *La potière jalouse*. Paris: Librairie Plon.
Lidz, T. and Lidz, R. W. (1989) *Oedipus in the Stone Age: A Psychoanalytic Study
of Masculinization in Papua New Guinea*. New York: International Universities
Press.
Matte-Blanco, I. (1975) *The Unconscious as Infinite Sets: An Essay in Bi-Logic*.
London: Duckworth.
—— (1988) *Thinking, Feeling, and Being: Clinical Reflections on the Funda-
mental Antinomy of Human Beings and World*. London and New York:
Routledge.
Moore, M. (1988) 'Mind, brain and unconscious', in P. Clark and C. Wright (eds)
Mind, Psycho- analysis and Science. Oxford: Blackwell.
Rayner, E. and Tuckett, D. (1988) 'An introduction to Matte-Blanco's reformu-
lation of the Freudian unconscious and his conceptualization of the internal
world', in I. Matte-Blanco, *Thinking, Feeling and Being*. London and New York:
Routledge.
—— and Wooster, G. (1990) 'Bi-logic in psychoanalysis and other disciplines: an
introduction', *International Review of Psycho-Analysis* 17: 425–31.
Segal, H. (1964) *Introduction to the Work of Melanie Klein*. London: The Hogarth
Press, rev. edn, 1973.
Steiner, J. (1985) 'Turning a blind eye: the cover up for Oedipus', *International
Review of Psycho-Analysis* 12: 161–72.
—— (1990) 'The retreat from truth to omnipotence in Sophocles' *Oedipus at
Colonus*', *International Review of Psycho-Analysis* 17: 227–37.

Index

Omaha kinship 42, 48
Omani 60, 62, 63
Orma 59
Ottenberg, S. 190

Paine, R. 82, 88
parricide 32, 33, 35, 37–8, 171, 202,
227, 233; in Australian myth 175–6,
177, 178, 228; in Bugisu 190, 203,
204, 230
participant observation *see*
anthropologist
person 19, 131–7, 146, 194, 203, 205;
gender and *see* gender, and identity;
Lacan and 147–50
phallus: feminist critique of Lacan's
phallocentrism 19, 20, 145, 148,
164; Gimi myth 217–18, 219, 236;
Lacanian psychoanalysis 146, 155,
157, 164–7, 195
phantasy 17, 115–25; applied to
working models 228–31, 232, 234;
and culture 23, 120–4, 198–9,
228–31, 232, 234, 236–7; defined
117; *see also* dreams; fantasy;
myth(s)
Pokomo 59
political 7, 167, 235; Gimi 234–5;
Islamic celebrations 15, 54–69, 235;
Oedipus myth 33, 35
polytheism 55, 66
post-structuralism 132, 135, 136
power relations 167; Islamic
celebrations 15, 54–69; Oedipus
myth 33, 35; *see also* gender
relations; political
pre-Oedipal *see* Oedipal stages of
development
primal father 21, 171, 202, 226–31
procreation beliefs 131, 140, 220–2,
237; Gimi 214–20, 232, 236–7;
Gisu 192–3, 201
psychoanalysis: as content 225–38;
diverse nature of 114–15, 124–5;
and dreams and unconscious
phantasy 115–24; relationship to
anthropology 1–24, 185, 222,
232–6 (*see also* complementarity;
ethnopsychoanalysis; *and under*
Lacan, Jacques)

psychoanalyst: difference in
methodology from anthropologist
18, 186, 204, 234

Quiche 102

Rainbow Serpent myth 174–8, 228,
229
reality: dream and 99–100; myth and
237
reciprocity 166; *see also* exchange
religion 123, 137, 187, 211, 231, 237;
Australian Aborigines 21, 176–7,
179–80, 181, 182, 206; and dreams
99; Freud and 202, 205; *see also*
Islam; myth(s); taboo(s)
Richards, A. 82, 83
Ricoeur, Paul 3, 30, 33, 35, 100, 160,
185, 186, 234
ritual 21, 123, 186–7; *see also* birth;
fertility; funerals; initiation;
marriage
Rosenfeld, Herbert 123

Sambian society 101
self 1, 4, 19, 90, 131–7, 144; Lacanian
143, 147–50, 154, 155, 160, 167;
see also gender, and identity; person
self-consciousness *see* knowledge
self-control, and Gisu circumcision
206–7, 230
Seligman, C.G. 2, 101
sexual identity, Lacan and 144–5,
147–8, 161, 164, 165
sexual symbolism: dancing 15, 67–9;
dreams 17, 102–3, 107, 108, 109;
Gisu circumcision 192–3, 231
sexuality 8, 9, 19, 131, 138, 139, 140,
143, 149, 150, 151; and dreams
101, 102–3, 106, 107, 108, 109; and
Gisu circumcision 185, 191–4, 195,
198, 202; Islamic 67–8; and
Newfoundland Young Yids 84, 91;
see also gender; homosexuality;
Oedipal stages of development
singing *see* dancing and singing
Smith, Jean 134
social constructionism 132, 133
social control 187, 206–7
socialisation: of aggression,